C000003305

# ABC OF MEDICAL COMPUTING

# ABC OF MEDICAL COMPUTING

Written and edited by

**NICHOLAS LEE** BSc MB BS FRCS FRCOphth
*Consultant Ophthalmologist, Western Eye and Hillingdon Hospitals (nicklee@nildram.co.uk)*

**ANDREW MILLMAN** MB BS DOccMed
*Occupational Physician, Nestlé UK Ltd, York (af89@dial.pipex.com)*

with contributions from

**ANDREW BROOKE,** *general practitioner, Gloucester*
**JOHN COX,** *head of information services, Wellcome Centre for Medical Science, London*
**ARA DARZI,** *consultant surgeon, minimal access surgery unit, St Mary's Hospital, London*
**KEVIN KEALY,** *Internet consultant, Unipalm PIPEX*
**SUE KINN,** *research fellow, Scottish Clinical Audit Research Centre, Glasgow University*
**HYLTON B MEIRE,** *consultant radiologist, Kings College Hospital, London*
**TERRY MORROW,** *BIDS marketing manager, University of Bath*
**MARTIN OSBORNE,** *senior registrar, Chase Farm Hospital, Enfield, Middlesex*
**JONATHAN POOLE,** *consultant occupational physician, Dudley Priority Health NHS Trust*
**JANE ROWLANDS,** *sublibrarian, BMA Library, BMA House, London*

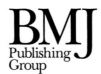

**BMJ**
Publishing
Group

© BMJ Publishing Group 1996

All rights reserved. No part of this publication may be reproduced, stored in a retrieval system, or transmitted, in any form or by any means, electronic, mechanical, photocopying, recording and/or otherwise, without the prior written permission of the publishers.

First published in 1996
by the BMJ Publishing Group, BMA House, Tavistock Square, London WC1H 9JR

**British Library Cataloguing in Publication Data**

A catalogue record for this book is available from the British Library

ISBN 0-7279-1046-9

Typeset by Apek Typesetters Ltd., Nailsea, Bristol
Printed by Clifford Press.

# CONTENTS

# PREFACE

Since the original *ABC of Medical Computing* was published in 1983, developments in information technology have advanced at an extraordinary pace matched only by the growth in the number of computers in daily use around the world. There can now be few health care professionals who do not regularly use a computer in one form or another but most have received precious little training in the use of modern computer systems and are often unable to get the best out of them. This book aims to address that need by taking the reader through the process of choosing, purchasing and setting up a computer, selecting and installing software and goes on to describe some common programs used in modern medicine.

For those already familiar with the basic principles, the book provides information about advanced concepts such as obtaining information from on-line resources and includes detailed guidance on the Internet and its relevance to medicine. Each chapter is heavily illustrated with photographs, diagrams and screen shots taken from working systems and includes a useful list of companies and organisations from whom you can obtain further information. Armed with this book, nobody need feel left behind or unable to make the most of their investment.

Nicholas Lee
Andrew Millman
*April 1996*

# ACKNOWLEDGMENTS

We would like to thank all the people who kindly read and made constructive comments about the text before publication. We are deeply indebted to the medical illustration departments at Gloucestershire Royal and Western Eye Hospitals who gave invaluable advice and practical help with some of the photographs we have used. We would also like to thank Malcolm Dees, Manager of IT Centre at Gloucestershire Royal Hospital for his advice about hospital computer systems, Roy Sharma, GP in Lydney, Gloucestershire for comments about the business aspects of GP computing, and Mr C Nduka, Research Fellow at St Mary's Hospital, for information about palmtop computers.

We would like to take this opportunity to thank our wives and families for their support and, not least, for giving us time to write this book.

The telephone numbers listed in this book are correct at the time of going to press.

# 1   AN INTRODUCTION TO COMPUTING IN MEDICAL PRACTICE

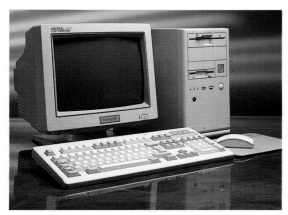

Modern desktop PC.

The past decade has seen an explosive growth in the number of computers, and in Britain alone there are now over 10 million in use. The capability of computers has also increased so that today's desktop PC is far more powerful than older main frame computers. This breathtaking pace of change has inevitably left many people behind. It is extraordinary that, despite the fact that information technology is now taught in every school, only a minority of current medical students consider themselves computer literate. The proportion of practising doctors who are able to get the best out of a computer is even smaller. We hope to remove some of the mystique from computing and to share our confidence that the technology can easily be mastered.

## What do computers have to offer?

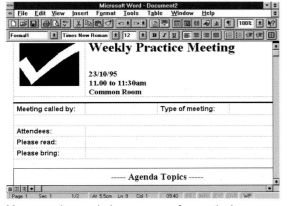

Most people use their computers for producing documents.

The commonest reason for buying a computer is the need to write simple letters, medical reports, papers, and curriculum vitae using a word processor. Most modern word processors are, however, capable of handling far more than simple text. You can create and incorporate colourful charts and graphics into your work. Many people will want to take this further and move on to desktop publishing in order to create complex documents such as practice leaflets. The best programs now incorporate a large number of blank templates to make the process as easy as possible.

## Managing data

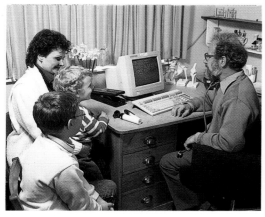

Using a general practice system.

Computers are good at storing and manipulating large amounts of information. Database programs collect, sort, and analyse this material, and perform repetitive tasks extremely fast and without error. Computers are also very accurate calculators and are thus able to carry out complex statistical analysis.

General practitioners have been quick to spot the potential benefits of computerising their practices. Several complex general practice systems are now available, all of which offer comprehensive recording of medical records, issue repeat prescriptions, and provide call and recall facilities. Many systems can also be linked to the local family health services authority and hospitals. There are add on programs to handle the inevitable administration, but many general practitioners use standard business software to manage the financial side of general practice.

# An introduction to computing in medical practice

## Slides

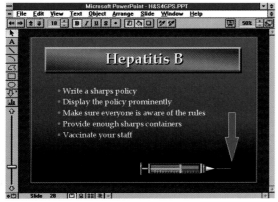

Slide produced on the computer.

At some time most doctors give presentations to colleagues or students. It is now easy to create eye catching slides or overhead transparencies on your computer, avoiding the need to rely on your medical illustration department. Furthermore, you can easily adapt slides created for past lectures, mix and match as required, and even change the appearance of every slide by pressing one key. Graphic images (clip art) and even photographs can be imported into your computer to make slides.

## Connection to others

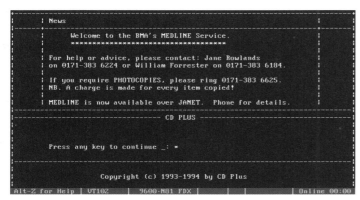

Medline search.

Connecting your computer to the public telephone system through a modem increases what you can do. It is easy to connect to and search remote databases such as Medline in the BMA's library. Most host systems allow you to transfer any information that you find over the telephone line into your own system. You can also transmit documents and data to colleagues anywhere in the world.

*Fax messages*

Sending fax messages directly from the computer has many advantages over conventional fax machines. Apart from being quicker, the text on the received fax is much clearer and therefore easier to read. Furthermore, the computer maintains a log of all faxes sent and received for future reference—electronic recorded delivery.

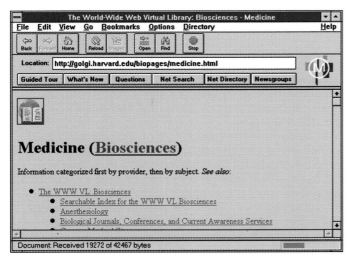

Surfing the Internet

*Internet*

The Internet has recently received a lot of publicity because the number of people connected to the system is growing rapidly. In addition to offering instantaneous email facilities, it is possible to link up with thousands of other computers on the system to get access to news, information, photographs, sound, or video on virtually any subject that you can imagine. Like it or not, computers are becoming increasingly integrated into our professional lives. Computers give us the ability to do tasks that were only dreamt of just a few decades ago and mastering them can help us to do our work faster and more efficiently.

# CD ROM

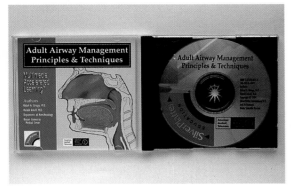

Multimedia programs are becoming more widely available.

CD ROMs (compact disc read only memory) have become increasingly popular in recent years. The discs, which are similar to the audio compact disc, are an excellent way of distributing large amounts of information and are easy to use. Basic discs contain simple text, but more complex multimedia discs contain a mixture of words, sound, pictures, and video. There are now many well produced medical titles for a range of health care professionals as well as for undergraduates. Some are almost unique reference sources for specialists working in a particular field.

# Networks

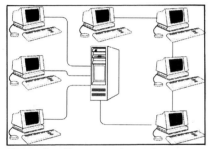

Networks allow users to pool resources.

Connecting computers to a network offers several important advantages. In most networks, confidential or important data are stored on a single central computer called a file server. This can be located in a secure environment, protecting the data from risks such as fire or theft. Access to the file server can be restricted to authorised users, further increasing security. Networks also allow users to work simultaneously, share resources such as printers and modems, and send electronic mail (email) to each other.

# 2 CHOOSING A COMPUTER SYSTEM

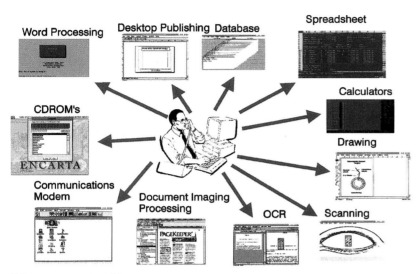

Word Processing · Desktop Publishing · Database · Spreadsheet · Calculators · Drawing · Scanning · OCR · Document Imaging Processing · Communications Modem · CDROM's · ENCARTA

What you can do with a computer.

Although computer equipment or hardware is continually falling in price, it represents a considerable investment and requires careful thought before purchase. Start by thinking what you wish the computer to do. Remember that you will probably soon find many unexpected uses for it and that the demands you place on the system are likely to grow. It is therefore important to buy a system that can be easily expanded and upgraded. Even the most basic computer will run a simple word processor, but a modern, user friendly graphical user interface such as Microsoft Windows requires a more powerful computer.

## IBM PC or Apple Macintosh?

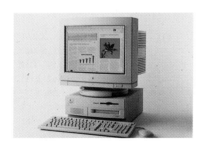

Apple Macintosh computer.

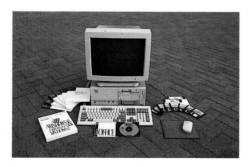

PC with a suite of software.

Many people are torn between buying an IBM PC and an Apple Macintosh. Both systems are excellent and have enthusiastic users. The Macintosh has been favoured because it has a graphical user interface which is easy to use and upgrading is simple. On the other hand, PCs now have a similar interface, are cheaper, and are more widely used. Furthermore, many companies offer optional extras for the PC at a reasonable price. Currently the PC dominates the business market while Macintosh has been favoured by graphic designers.

An extensive range of software is available for both formats, and most of the major programs are now available for both the PC and Macintosh. There is also a trend towards common file formats so that work can easily be transferred from one to the other. It is often best to buy the same type of computer as used in your department because there will be an established body of expertise to draw on and you will be able to share resources with your colleagues. As most people use PCs we have focused on these, but the basic principles can be applied to both types of hardware.

In some ways computers are like modular hi-fi systems—you can choose from a wide range of components of variable specification and price. This allows great flexibility but can be rather daunting. We have suggested some minimum specifications, but you should talk to suppliers to become familiar with the options and the terminology. The simplest option is to buy a complete package off the shelf. You can expect to get a good combination of basic hardware and sometimes a suite of software at no extra cost. It is simple to add or replace individual parts of the system at a later date—unlike other items of electrical equipment, computers have been designed to be easily upgraded.

# Central processing unit (cpu)

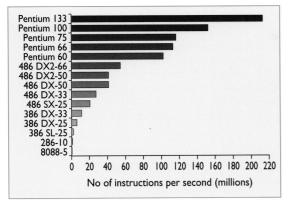

No of instructions per second (millions)

Relative performance of processors.

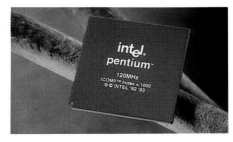

Intel Pentium processor.

Computers are driven by a microprocessor chip. IBM chose a chip manufactured by Intel for the original PC first sold in 1982. Since then, Intel has continued to develop the processor, and there has been a steady increase in the power and capability of the PC as a result. Today's computer bears little resemblance to the original PC, but it will still run early programs.

You will sometimes see a DX2 or DX4 suffix after a chip number. These chips run two to four times faster internally while still communicating with the rest of the computer at a standard speed and offer substantial performance gains without the cost of modifying the rest of the system.

The Intel Pentium is the latest generation of chip and runs faster than the 486. If you are on a tight budget the 486 processor offers excellent value for money. At the time of going to press, the pentium 75 is the entry level processor but it is certain to be superseded very rapidly. However, leading edge technology always carries a price premium, and it is sometimes better to choose an older, cheaper chip with a view to upgrading later when the price has fallen.

The motherboard, on which the processor sits, is also important. Modern high specification boards include built in interfaces for devices such as hard disks and hard disk modems, saving the need to buy extra expansion cards. Some also include high quality stereo sound cards. The latest motherboards include energy saving features that automatically power down the whole computer after a period of inactivity. "Plug and play" systems automatically recognise and configure additional components such as modems, sound cards, CD ROMs, and printers, which greatly simplifies installation.

# Random Access Memory (RAM)

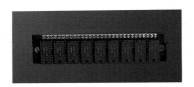

SIMM (single inline memory module).

All computers need electronic working space in which to perform calculations, draw graphics, etc. Complex work demands more space. The working memory or RAM can be accessed almost instantly, but all the information held in RAM is lost when the computer is switched off. The size of a computer's memory is expressed in megabytes. Most standard computers are sold with 4 megabytes of RAM. If you wish to run Windows, increasing the memory to 8 Mb greatly improves the computer's performance, while 16 Mb is recommended for those using Windows 95.

# Hard disk

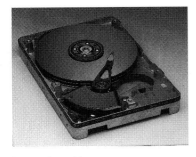

Internal workings
of hard disk.

The hard disk is used to store programs and data and is the electronic equivalent of a filing cabinet. Even though modern hard disks store considerable amounts of information, they tend to fill up very rapidly. This is partly due to the increasing size of modern software. For example, some Windows programs can use as much as 20 to 30 Mb each. You should therefore buy the largest hard disk that you can afford and not consider anything much smaller than 300 Mb. Fortunately, the price of large hard disks has fallen considerably in recent years, and it is possible to double a disk's capacity safely with disk compression software.

## System box

> ### Optional extras for the computer
>
> *CD ROM drive*—Offers access to a wealth of information
> *Sound card*—Required for multimedia CD ROMs
> *Tape streamer*—Most common backup system
> *Fax modem*—For communicating with the outside world
> *Scanner*—To copy photographs, diagrams, etc into the computer
> *Network card*—To connect to the office network

You will need to decide which case best meets your needs. A small case occupies less space but does not leave much room for additional components if you decide to upgrade. If desk space is at a premium, the system box could be placed on the floor, although this can be inconvenient as the case contains the floppy disk drive. If you are planning an expanding system, a free standing tower case is a good choice.

## Monitor or visual display unit

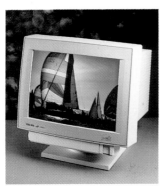

A non-flickering (super VGA) colour monitor puts less strain on your eyes.

Since you will spend many hours working at the computer, it is worth taking time to find a good monitor. Most visual display units measure 14" (35 cm), but many companies now offer a 15" (38 cm) screen for a small premium. It is often a price worth paying. Those planning to create numerous complex graphics should consider a 17" (43 cm) screen, although these are much more expensive. Choose a super video graphics array (super VGA) monitor capable of running in non-interlaced mode to avoid screen flicker.

The video card is an important component of the computer; it collects digital signals from the processor and drives the screen. Graphical user interfaces are complex and require a good video card in order to process the large volume of visual information. Many modern video cards are connected to the computer by a fast electronic channel called a local bus, which considerably enhances performance: PCI is now the dominant standard. Several accelerated video cards are also available, which make Windows software run faster.

## Portable computers

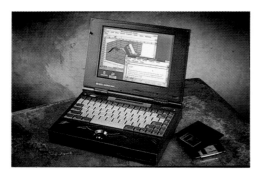

Hewlett Packard Notebook.

> ### Points to consider when buying a portable computer
>
> *Keyboard*—Feel; size of shift and return keys
> *Mouse position and ease of use*—Can it get lost?
> *Screen*—Monochrome or colour
> *Battery*—Check battery life and replacement costs
> *Construction*—Does it feel robust?
> *PCMCIA*—Allows the use of many accessories
> *Insurance*—Portables are more prone to damage and theft

The performance of current portable computers is little different from that of the desktop computer. When size and portability are paramount portable computers are ideal; otherwise, a desktop computer is a better choice as it is much more robust and versatile. Portable computers are much more expensive than desktops.

Choosing a portable is more difficult than choosing a desktop as there are more factors to consider. Unlike desktop computers the keyboard, mouse, and screen vary enormously. It is important to try several portables before you buy to ensure that you are comfortable with your final choice.

*Screens and batteries*

Until recently monochrome liquid crystal displays (LCD) were almost ubiquitous on portable computers. However, manufacturers now offer excellent colour screens. Monochrome screens are cheaper but, unless your budget is limited, the extra expense is easily justified. There are two types of colour screen, the DualScan (D-STN), which offers a good balance between performance and cost, and the thin film transistor (TFT), which is better but more expensive.

Portable computers will run continuously for about two hours between charges. Many now offer built in power saving features which extend battery life considerably.

*Expansion*

Most modern portable computers have at least one PCMCIA (Personal Computer Memory Card International Association) slot to allow connection of external components—for example, fax modem, network card, or hard disk. Most also have sockets for plugging in a standard colour monitor, keyboard, or mouse. A few portables have a built in CD ROM drive, but most need to be connected to an external drive.

# Printers

### Types of printers

| Monochrome | Colour |
| --- | --- |
| Dot matrix | Colour inkjet |
| Inkjet | Wax thermal transfer |
| Laser printer | Colour laser printer |
| | Dye sublimination |

The final quality of your documents depends on the output from your printer. Even very old computers can drive the latest laser printer to produce polished pages. As with other parts of the system, you will need to balance print quality against the cost of a printer and its running costs.

A laser printer produces the highest quality output, although until recently they have been relatively expensive both to buy and to run. However, users of Windows can take advantage of cheap GDI laser printers. Inkjet printers are smaller, quieter, and cheaper, although running costs are about the same as a laser. Inkjet print quality is not quite as good as that from a laser but is more than adequate for routine correspondence. Inkjets can also print pictures and charts, and colour versions are reasonably priced.

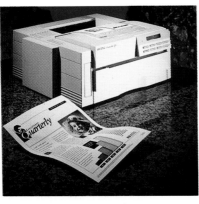

Hewlett Packard laser printer.

Dot matrix printers are the cheapest, but their print quality is poor and they are very noisy. Dot matrix printers are, however, well suited to printing on tractor feed paper and multipart forms. Another advantage of dot matrix printers is that ink is impregnated into the paper. It is therefore more permanent than laser printed text, which simply sticks to the surface of the paper. This may be important for medicolegal reasons.

All printers can print on to A4 paper, but you should also ask whether the printer you are considering is capable of printing on to acetate sheets for overhead presentations and on to different sizes of paper. Many general practitioners prefer letters printed on A5 rather than A4 paper as A5 fits more easily into standard records. Users of portable computers may wish to consider a compact battery operated printer which allows printing on the move. Before choosing a printer ask to see an example of its print quality and compare this with samples from other makes.

# Manufacturer

### Manufacturers of computers and printers

*Computers*
| | |
| --- | --- |
| Apple Macintosh | 0800 127753 |
| Compaq | 0990 134456 |
| Compusys | 01296 395531 |
| Dan | 0181 830 1100 |
| Dell | 01344 720000 |
| Elonex | 0181 452 4444 |
| Evesham Micros | 01386 765500 |
| Gateway | 0800 602000 |
| IBM | 0990 426426 |
| Taxan Monitors | 01344 484646 |
| Viglen | 0181 758 7000 |

*Printers*
| | |
| --- | --- |
| Brother | 0345 535100 |
| Cannon | 0800 252223 |
| Epson | 0800 220456 |
| Hewlett Packard | 01344 369222 |
| Star | 01494 471111 |
| Kodak | 01442 61122 |

Choosing an established manufacturer is important because many computer companies have gone into liquidation in recent years. Computer equipment is generally very reliable but is eventually likely to need attention. We therefore recommend that you buy from a reputable company. Most manufacturers have showrooms where you can try their computers before purchase. If you decide to use mail order, always purchase goods costing more than £100 with a credit card as this protects you against bankruptcy of the supplier.

# 3   UNDERSTANDING YOUR COMPUTER

At first sight desktop computers seem very complex, but they are really quite simple. Understanding the purpose of each component and the way that they are put together will help you get the best from your system.

## External features

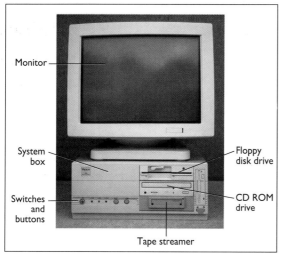

PC with a standard desktop case.

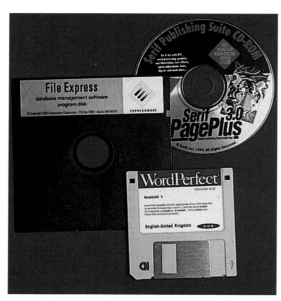

Different types of disk.

*Monitor*

By default video graphics array (VGA) monitors run at a resolution of $640 \times 480$ pixels (dots) on the screen. Super VGA monitors can be set to run at higher resolutions—for example, $800 \times 600$ or $1024 \times 768$. These resolutions allow more detail to be displayed on the screen, although text may become too small to read comfortably on a standard 14″ monitor. Higher resolutions are therefore best used on larger screens.

*System box*

This houses all the main components of the computer such as the motherboard, processor, memory, and hard disk as well as all the expansion cards and optional extras—for example, the CD ROM drive.

*Switches and buttons*

*Keyboard lock*—A key operated switch which disables the keyboard. Not as useful as it seems because the keys are often interchangeable.

*Reset button*—This switch instantly restarts the computer, which can be useful if a program locks for any reason. Pushing the button accidentally will result in permanent loss of all unsaved work.

*Turbo*—Far from speeding things up, this button actually slows the computer down. It is provided because some very old programs will not run at high speed but is rarely needed or used.

*Floppy drive*

Floppy disks are used to transfer information and programs into and out of a computer. Older $5\frac{1}{4}$″ disks were literally flexible and vulnerable to damage. Modern $3\frac{1}{2}$″ disks have a hard plastic case that protects them. Standard double sided high density floppy disks can store up to 1.44 megabytes of information.

Before a floppy disk can be used it has to be formatted—a process in which the disk is divided into segments which the computer uses to store data. All computers can format disks, although each disk takes a minute or more. You can buy preformatted disks but these are more expensive.

*CD ROM drive*

This drive is used to read all types of CD ROM (compact disc read only memory). Many suites of programs such as Microsoft Office are now provided on CD ROM as these would otherwise have to be supplied on a large number of floppy disks. The CD ROM drive in the figure is mounted in a $5\frac{1}{4}$″ drive bay, which could also be used for a tape streamer.

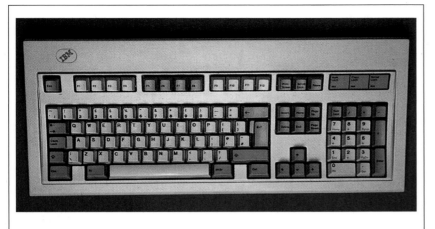

| | |
|---|---|
| Alt key | This selects an alternative function. For example, in windows programs holding down the Alt key and then pressing E (often written as Alt-E) activates the edit menu rather than putting the letter E on the page |
| Ctrl key | The control key is used in a similar way to the Alt key. For example, in Windows Ctrl-P prints the document |
| Esc key | Pressing escape usually cancels a selection or exits from a programme |
| F1 to F12 | Function keys are used to select specific functions. For example, pressing F10 in Word-perfect for DOS saves the document |
| ↑ ← | The arrow keys move the cursor around the screen |
| Insert | Toggles between typeover and insert mode. In typeover mode new characters overwrite those on the screen whereas in insert mode they are inserted into the text |
| Home | Used in combination with arrow keys to move cursor to top of the page, beginning of the line, etc |
| Page up & page down | Move the cursor up and down one page at a time |
| End | Moves cursor to end of the line |
| Delete | Deletes characters to the right of the cursor |
| Backspace | Deletes characters to the left of the cursor |
| Numeric keypad | Fast and convenient way of entering numbers. the four basic arithmetic functions are on the surrounding keys |
| ↵ | The carriage return and enter keys are completely interchangeable |

The keyboard.

### Mouse

A mouse is essential for controlling graphical user interfaces such as Windows. The mouse contains a rolling ball, and moving across the desk moves an arrow shaped pointer around the screen. Most have two buttons. The left button is normally used to select or activate any object that you point to. Clicking the right button usually brings up a function menu.

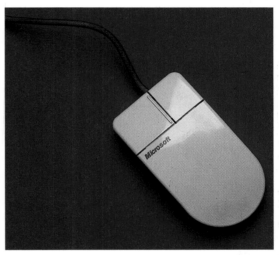

The mouse.

## Inside the computer

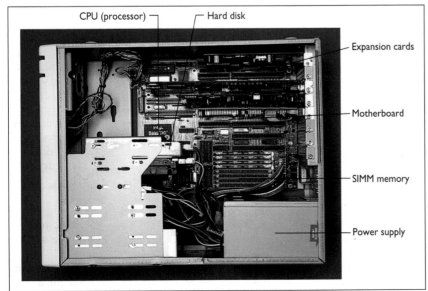

Inside of a computer.

*Motherboard*—This is the main circuit board on to which other parts of the computer are attached.

*Processor*—This is the heart of the computer (see page 5).

*Memory or RAM*—Computers use single in-line memory modules which plug into sockets on the motherboard. Additional modules can easily be inserted into empty sockets. They are available in both 32 and 72 pin versions, which are not interchangeable.

*Hard disk*—An essential part of the computer where programs are stored. Hard disks have far greater capacity and work much faster than floppy disks. When your hard disk is full, an additional hard disk can be added or disk compression software used to pack more data into your existing hard disk.

## Understanding your computer

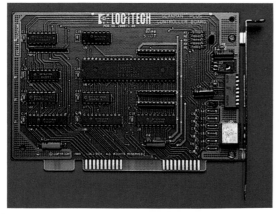

Expansion card.

*Expansion cards*—These are used to connect the motherboard to essential peripherals (hard and floppy disk drives, serial and parallel ports, and the monitor) and to optional extras (CD ROM drive, modem, tape streamer, sound card, or scanner). It is very easy to plug additional expansion cards into free sockets.

*Speaker*—The standard internal speaker is adequate for warning bleeps and simple tones. To listen to more sophisticated sound, such as speech and music (which are an essential part of multimedia), you will need to install a sound card and hi-fi speakers containing a built in, mains powered stereo amplifier.

## Back of the computer

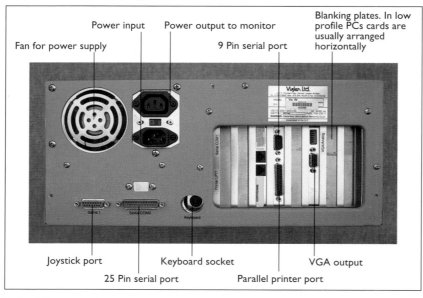

Back of the computer.

*Fan*—Noisy but essential to keep the inside of the computer cool.

*Power*—The mains lead plugs into one socket. The other similar looking socket supplies switched mains power from the computer to the monitor so that there is no need to switch off the monitor each time you turn off the computer.

*VGA output*—Connect the monitor here.

*Serial port*—There are usually two serial sockets, which can have either 9 or 25 pins. One is used for the mouse. The other can be used to connect an external modem or to link two computers using a null modem cable.

*Parallel port*—Most computers have just one parallel port, which is used to connect the computer to the printer.

*Keyboard socket*—5 pin DIN socket used for the keyboard.

Removing the lid of your computer does not invalidate the guarantee, as is the case with much electrical equipment.

## Operating systems

### Drive labels

A:\    First floppy drive
B:\    Second floppy drive if installed
C:\    Main hard disk
D:\  ⎫ Further letters are used for
E:\  ⎬ additional hard disks, RAM disk,
F:\  ⎭ CD ROM drive, or network drive

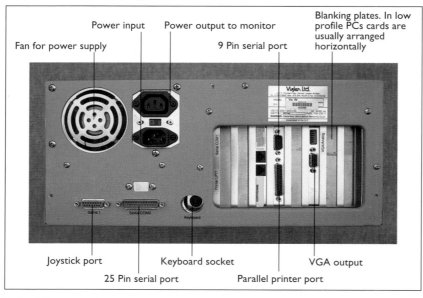

Windows 95 has a brand new, easy to use, graphical interface.

When the computer is turned on, it automatically runs a series of tests to ensure that all its components are plugged in and working properly. Once this has been completed it loads the operating system from the first track of the hard disk (known as the boot sector) into memory. This process is known as booting up. The operating system controls the computer and translates commands that you issue in English (such as save or print) into instructions which drive the hardware. Almost all computers are supplied with an operating system known as MS DOS (Microsoft disk operating system), although there are many others. They include:

*Windows*—Optional extra, which sits on top of DOS and provides a friendly graphical interface to the user.

*Windows 95*—New version of Windows which does not need DOS and is designed to take full advantage of modern processors.

*Windows NT*—Completely new, and highly advanced and secure 32 bit operating system aimed at a few specialised corporate applications rather than ordinary users.

*IBM OS/2 Warp*—Modern operating system sold by IBM which is similar to Windows 95. It can run DOS and Windows programs as well as software specifically written for OS/2.

*Unix*—Modern 32 bit operating system which allows several people to work on the same computer simultaneously. Many general practice systems are based on it.

The operating system is usually installed by the manufacturer.

## Filenames

Filenames take the format of up to eight characters with a full stop separating a three character extension. The filename extension gives useful information on the nature of the file.

*EXE, *.COM, and *.BAT indicate files that will run programs

*DOC, *.TXT, and *.WRI are typical document file extensions

*PXC, *.TIF, and *.BMP are extensions for bit mapped graphic files

## Useful DOS commands

| | |
|---|---|
| A: | Change the prompt to the A or floppy drive |
| CD | Change directory—for example, CD MS DOS will change you into the MS DOS directory |
| CD \ | Changes you back to the root directory |
| Copy SUMMARY.DOC A: | Copies the file SUMMARY.DOC to the floppy disk in drive A |
| DEL SUMMARY.DOC | Deletes the file SUMMARY.DOC |
| DIR/P | Lists the directories and files one page at a time |
| Format A: | Formats the floppy disk in drive A |
| Help | Displays a help menu giving all available MS DOS commands and instructions on how to use them |
| MD | Make a new directory—for example, MD LETTERS would create a directory called LETTERS |
| RD | Remove a directory |
| UNDELETE | Restores a previously deleted file |

*Configuration files*

As the operating system is loading the computer reads two special configuration files called AUTOEXEC.BAT and CONFIG.SYS which tell the computer how to set itself up. During the boot process you will see a lot of rapidly scrolling text on the screen as each of the commands in these configuration files are carried out. This text can usually be ignored. Experienced users sometimes modify configuration files to optimise the operation of the computer. Beginners are advised to leave them alone since errors in these files can result in the computer failing to start. When the computer has finished booting many computers simply display the prompt (C: >) until you enter a command. Others will automatically run a menu or proceed directly into Windows.

At this stage the computer is ready to use. This is the best time to organise your hard disk (see page 80). The computer may have come with software already installed, or you may now need to choose which software you are going to buy and use. If the software is installed typing the initial command—for example, win for Windows, wp for WordPerfect—will start it running.

# 4 CHOOSING AND INSTALLING SOFTWARE

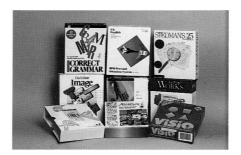

Examples of modern software.

All computers, no matter how sophisticated, need programs or software to be able to complete the simplest task. Programs provide not only the functions that we have come to expect from modern computer systems but also the interface between you and the computer hardware. There is a huge range of software on the market, and choosing the program that best meets your needs can sometimes be difficult. A useful point to remember is that well designed programs allow you to complete complex tasks easily and quickly. Having the right program often saves hours of work. This chapter concentrates on software for stand alone computers; software for general practices and for networks is covered later.

## What type of software?

---

**Type of software to buy**

| Task | Software |
| --- | --- |
| Letter writing | Simple word processor |
| Creating posters, handouts, leaflets, books | Graphic user interface word processor or desktop publishing |
| Diary, address book | Personal information managers |
| Making slides or charts | Presentation software |
| Creating diagrams | Graphics software |
| Using ready prepared images | Clip art library |
| Storing or retrieving information | Databases |
| Managing references | Bibliographic software |
| Data manipulation or budget planning | Spreadsheets |
| Statistical analysis | Statistics software |
| Practice accounts | Accounting software |
| Accessing Medline, Internet, etc | Communication software |
| Housekeeping | Utilities programs |

---

*Category of software*

First identify which type of software would be most appropriate for the task. In most cases the category of software needed is obvious, although the distinction between advanced word processors and desktop publishing programs has become somewhat blurred.

*DOS or Windows?*

Most programs are available in both DOS and Windows versions. Many organisations, including the NHS, have a large number of old computers that can run only DOS based programs. For simple letter writing and accessing the patient administration system (PAS), these older computers are more than adequate. Given the increased capabilities and user friendliness of Windows, however, most people with modern computers are moving to Windows based software.

---

**Suites of programs**

*Works suites*
- Microsoft Works
- Perfect Works
- Lotus Works
- Claris Works
- IBM Works

*Office suites*
- Corel Office Professional—WordPerfect, Quattro Pro, Presentations, Paradox
- Microsoft Office—Word, Excel, Powerpoint, Access
- Lotus SmartSuite—AmiPro, Lotus 1-2-3, Freelance Graphics, Approach

---

*Stand alone program or suites*

People often buy a single program such as WordPerfect, but it makes sense to consider one of the software suites. These integrated packages include all the basic programs—word processor, spreadsheet, presentation graphics, and database—and may also include other useful software. The programs in a suite have the advantage of a common look and feel and will have been designed to work well together. They also represent very good value for money compared with buying each of the programs separately. The basic "Works" suites offer all the features most people need and cost less than £100. If you want very comprehensive facilities you should buy one of the "Office" suites, but these are more expensive. Suites do not include specialist applications such as programs for statistical analysis, which have to be purchased separately. Many computers are sold with a suite of software, which may tip the balance in favour of one type of computer.

## Information sources about software

Software reviews in computer magazines
Computer dealers
Computer exhibitions
Online services (Internet, CompuServe)
Information leaflets or demonstration disks
   from manufacturer
Demonstration or recommendation from a
   colleague
National Information on Software and
   Services (01225 826176)

*Selecting the individual program*

Many people worry about the benefits of one program over another, but the main programs have now evolved to the point where they have all the features most people are likely to need. The choice boils down to personal or departmental preference. Computer magazines regularly publish comparisons of programs, which give some indication of their relative features and merit. However, the best way of making sure that the software meets your needs is to try it.

# Shareware and public domain programs

## Types of software

| | |
|---|---|
| Public domain | No licence required |
| Shareware | Free trial period, buy licence later |
| Commercial | Purchase licence immediately |

As well as commercial programs, you might like to consider using Shareware. This is essentially a different way of marketing software in which you are able to install and use a program free of charge for a limited period. If, after this, you decide to continue using the software you have to pay for it. Shareware programs can be obtained from Shareware libraries, which advertise in computer magazines, or can be down loaded from a bulletin board using a modem. The quality of Shareware programs varies, but many are at least as good as their commercial counterparts.

# Where to buy from

## Where to buy from

Computer dealers
High street stores
Computer supermarkets
Mail order
Direct from manufacturer or supplier
Combined Higher Education Software Team
   (01225 826176)
Hospital or medical school suppliers

The computer market is fiercely competitive, and it is always worth comparing prices before buying a program. Advice and support from your local dealer can be invaluable even if you have to pay slightly more for the software. The mail order firms advertising in computer magazines are usually cheapest, but remember that fierce competition does lead to companies going out of business.

*Look for a discount*

Many software companies offer discounts for those working at academic, educational, or health care institutions, so always check to see if you might be eligible. It is best to contact the companies directly for details as many dealers are unaware of these special offers. Software or hardware purchased by a charitable trust is usually exempt from value added tax, but remember that the product then remains the property of the trust. This method should not be used for making personal purchases. If you need to upgrade from a simple to a complex program many companies offer attractive competitive trade up discounts.

## Safeguarding your purchase

- Get a written quote
- Keep a record of your order
- Credit cards offer protection for purchases over £100
- Some magazines support the Mail Order Protection Scheme (MOPS)
- Consider paying cash on delivery

*Academic institutions*

CHEST (Combined Higher Education Software Team), an organisation funded by the universities and research councils, makes commercial software available to the higher education community at large discounts. Further details are contained in the CHEST book (published by Bath University Press). People with access to the joint academic network (JANET) can also obtain up to date online information from National Information on Software and Services, including the latest version of the CHEST software directory.

# Software updates

All programs are regularly revised and improved and then released with a higher version number. These updated programs invariably contain many new features which may or may not be useful to you. Updates should therefore be judged on their merits, but users of Windows 95 should seriously consider new, 32 bit versions of older software.

## Loading programs

### Copying installation disks

Open the write protection tab to ensure the computer does not accidentally write to your master disks

**DOS**
At the C\prompt type:
   Diskcopy a: a:
Insert the source (original) disk as directed
Insert a formatted destination disk as directed

**Windows 95**
Double click on My Computer
Single click on drive containing source disk
From the file menu, click copy disk
Click start

Source disk=Disk you are copying
Destination disk=Blank formatted disk

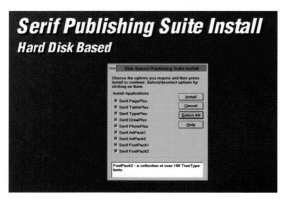

Options for installing Serif software.

Software is distributed on floppy disks or CD ROM and will need to be loaded on to the computer. Before you do this take a few minutes to read the manual, which will contain detailed instructions. Because original installation disks are valuable and can and do get damaged, we recommend that you make a set of back up disks and use these instead of the originals.

You usually start running an install or setup program on the first floppy disk. This will automatically copy the program to the computer and configure it for use.

Most modern programs are modular. In many cases you are offered a choice of full installation (which installs every module), custom install (which allows you to select the modules you want to install), and minimum installation (which installs only those parts of the program which are essential for it to run properly). The last option is useful if you are short of hard disk space, but you will lose some features.

Many modern programs are supplied on either floppy disk or CD ROM. The latter offer many advantages including speed and ease of installation. They are also more robust, and often include extras such as full online manuals and additional clip art or fonts. Some programs can be run wholly or partly from the CD ROM. This saves hard disk space, but programs will then take longer to load and may run more slowly.

## Starting the program

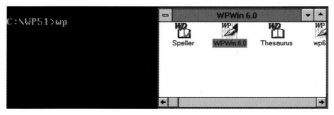

Starting WordPerfect in DOS and Windows.

For DOS based programs the manual will indicate what to type at the DOS prompt—for example, WP for WordPerfect, SC5 for SuperCalc spreadsheet. For Windows programs you have to point to the program icon with the mouse and double click with the left mouse button.

## Software registration

**Warning: This computer program is protected by copyright law and international treaties. Unauthorised reproduction or distribution of this program, or any portion of it, may result in severe civil and criminal penalities, and will be prosecuted to the maximum extent possible under the law.**

OK

Breaching copyright can lead to serious penalties

Do not forget to register your software as this will entitle you to technical support and discounts on future upgrades. Software is usually licensed to be installed on only one computer. Some companies will allow users to install programs on a portable or home computer as well as the work computer providing that it is used on only one computer at a time. Check your licence agreement first. Sharing software is illegal, and in many hospitals the use of pirated software is a disciplinary offence. The Federation Against Software Theft (FAST) has been set up to track down users of illegitimate software and has made unannounced visits to NHS premises. In any event it is a false economy to use pirated software as you will never get the best out of the program without the manuals or technical support.

### Advantages and disadvantages of DOS based and Windows programs

**DOS based**

*Advantages*
Simple and occupy less disk space than Windows based programs
Ideal for basic tasks such as letter writing
Run quickly on older computers
Text easy to read on standard monitor
Stable and rarely crash

*Disadvantages*
No consistent look and feel to programs
Transferring information between programs is more difficult
Not easy to judge page layout
Cannot view graphics
All text looks the same on the screen (no matter what typeface or size)

**Windows based**

*Advantages*
Attractive, user friendly interface
Consistent feel and look to programs
WYSIWYG screen—what you see is what you get
View colour pictures and text simultaneously
Can run several programs simultaneously
Easy to cut and paste between programs
Printer, fax modem, fonts, etc available to all programs
Comprehensive online help is always available

*Disadvantages*
Slow on older computers
Programs are often very large
Requires more sophisticated hardware
More liable to crash

# Getting help

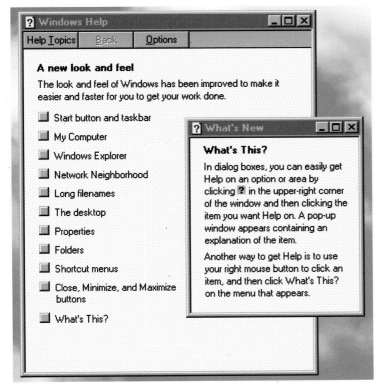

Windows 95 contains extensive help screens.

Most programs are supplied with manuals which should be read before using the program. There is an increasing trend to reduce the size of the manuals and provide this information in the form of help screens on the computer. The help screens not only contain information normally found in the manual, but, with Windows 95, there are hypertext links between pages and active buttons that run additional programs which can take you through your problem step by step. If you cannot find the answer to your query using the information supplied contact the manufacturer of the software for technical support by telephone, fax, or email.

# 5   GETTING YOUR THOUGHTS ON PAPER

| Advantages of word processors |
|---|
| Text is fully editable |
| Work can be saved and stored |
| Documents look professional |
| Writing tools such as spell checker |
| Mail merging |
| Macros for doing repetitive tasks |
| Automatic indexing |
| Graphics, spreadsheets, and charts |

Word processing is almost always the first facility people use on the computer, and for many people it is the main reason for buying a computer. The tremendous flexibility of even the most basic word processors has ensured that they have almost totally replaced the typewriter. Word processors allow you to create and then amend parts of the document before printing so that you never have to retype the whole document.

## Document display

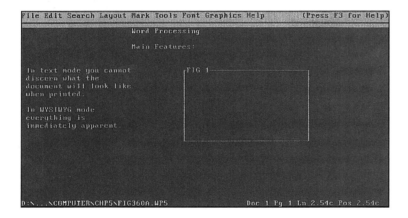

Until recently, most business word processing has been done with DOS based programs that use character based screens. These programs load, run, and print quickly even on old computers but have the disadvantage that you cannot see exactly what the page will look like when printed without switching to a preview screen. However, newer programs have moved to graphical screens with a WYSIWYG display (what you see is what you get). This means that you see exactly what the printed page will look like as you type it, which is invaluable with more complex documents.

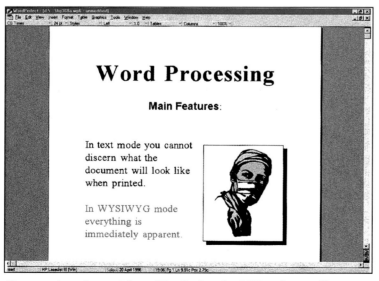

Typing is a keyboard activity, and all word processors allow functions to be selected by pressing various keys. This is both a strength and a weakness. Once you have learnt the key strokes of a particular program most people are reluctant to learn new ones. The Windows environment is starting to introduce uniformity between programs, with the same key strokes performing the same action. The mouse pointing device, which is used with Windows and other graphical interfaces, is used to simplify adjustments to the page and to duplicate control of many standard functions. Although it is easier to learn to use, the keyboard is usually quicker.

Character based screen from WordPerfect for DOS and same file on a graphical screen with WYSIWYG display.

# Moving text

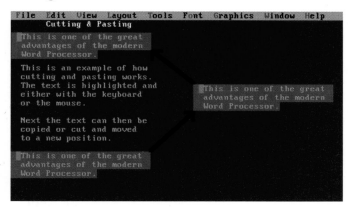

Text is easily moved by cutting and pasting.

An important advantage of a word processor over a typewriter is the ability to move blocks of text around a document or to cut text from other documents and paste it into the current document. This is performed by blocking an area of text, copying or cutting the block, and then moving it to the document in which you wish to insert the text and pasting it in. Many word processors now allow several documents to be open at once, which is a big help when cutting and pasting.

# Choosing the typeface

```
Monspaced typewriter font (courier)
```
Proportionally spaced serif font (eg. Times Roman)
**Proportionally spaced sans serif font (eg. Univers)**
**Modern Artistic typeface (eg. Britannic bold)**
𝕿𝖗𝖆𝖉𝖎𝖙𝖎𝖔𝖓𝖆𝖑 𝖈𝖆𝖑𝖑𝖎𝖌𝖗𝖆𝖕𝖍𝖎𝖈 𝖋𝖔𝖓𝖙 (eg. 𝕺𝖑𝖉𝖊 𝕰𝖓𝖌𝖑𝖎𝖘𝖍)
Bold, *Italic* and <u>Underline</u>
Different point sizes (8, 12, 16, 20, 24)

**White on black background**

**Coloured text (colour printers only)**

Most word processors allow you to choose which typeface or font that you want to use in your document. The old Courier monospaced font used by typewriters is much more difficult to read than proportionally spaced fonts. There are over 20 000 different fonts available from font libraries, but the two most used are Times Roman and Universal. A different font increases the impact of newsletters, handouts, posters, invitations, etc. In the Windows environment all programs share a common font pool enabling fonts supplied with one program to be used by any other program. You can also change the appearance of a font by using features such as bold, italic, and underline.

# Tables and graphics

The table facility allows you to create a grid into which you can precisely place text, numbers, or graphics. The more advanced tables have over 100 powerful spreadsheet functions enabling complex calculations to be performed on the data. You can also import data from other spreadsheet programs or databases. It is often easier to process data with a spreadsheet program, but a word processor is far more flexible for printing out the report on the data. Once you have created a table it is easy to adjust the style or even sort the data alphabetically.

| Column A<br>Row 1 | Column B<br>No used | Column C<br>Cost/item<br>(pence) | Column D<br>Total cost<br>(pence) |
|---|---|---|---|
| Row 2<br>Needles | 10 | 5 | (B2 * C2)<br>50 |
| Row 3<br>Syringes | 10 | 20 | (B3 * C3)<br>200 |
| Row 4<br>Swabs | 3 | 150 | (B4 * C4)<br>450 |
| Row 5<br>Total | +(symbol<br>for summing<br>column)<br>23 | +<br><br>175 | +<br><br>700 |

Table created with a word processor.

Adding a graphic image can increase the impact of your document. To do this you need to create a box into which the picture is placed. Most word processors allow images to be imported from a variety of other drawing programs. Windows word processors also have basic drawing tools available and can import images from a scanner.

# Useful tools

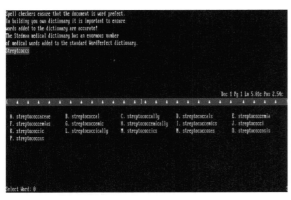

Spell checkers can have medical dictionaries added.

### Spell checkers

Undoubtedly the most useful accessory is a spell checker. Though the larger dictionaries have over 100 000 words that include the basic medical words, most medical terminology will not be included. Individual new words can be inserted in the dictionary, and *Stedman's Medical Dictionary* can replace the main WordPerfect dictionary. This provides over 165 000 additional medical words including medical procedures, devices, diseases, drug names, acronyms, and abbreviations. A spell checker will not identify the use of an incorrect but correctly spelt word, such as "too" instead of "to" or the absence of a full stop. A grammar checker can analyse and suggest corrections for such errors. The thesaurus is also useful.

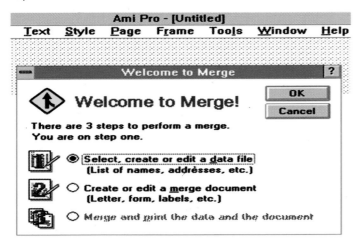

Merge facilities allow you to personalise mass mailing.

### Macros

You will often need a particular phrase such as "Kind regards" or "Yours sincerely" time and time again. This can be simplified by creating a macro which inserts the text automatically. The macro recorder memorises a sequence of keystrokes and allows you to play them back at will by pressing a simple combination of keys such as Alt K or Ctrl Y. The recording facility can also be used to simplify the creation of complex documents such as letters and discharge summaries. Those willing to spend time learning the macro language will be able to add very powerful features to their word processor.

# Importing and exporting files

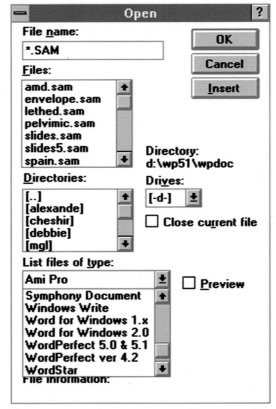

Most programs allow you to open files saved with different packages.

### Export and import filters

Unfortunately all programs save files in different formats. For example, to use work created in WordPerfect on another computer running Word you have to save on to a floppy disk and then import it with the WordPerfect filter of Word. Most word processing packages have an extensive range of export and import filters, and you can usually find a common file format for transfer. Exchanging data between PCs and Apple computers is also possible.

### Faxes

Adding a fax modem to your computer allows you to send a document that you have created on the screen to fax machines anywhere in the world moments after you have finished typing. The quality of faxes sent in this way is better than those that are sent with a standard fax machine.

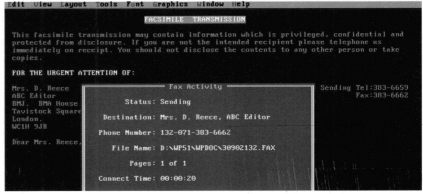

Sending a fax from within WordPerfect

# Speech recognition

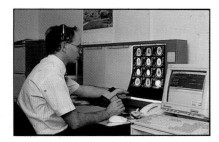

Using a speech recognition system.

Speech recognition allows you to dictate text directly into the computer at speeds of over 100 words per minute. The whole computer can be controlled by voice so that it is hardly necessary to touch the keyboard.

There are currently three different types of speech recognition system. The Dragon Dictate system recognises individual words, which are dictated directly into standard Windows applications such as WordPerfect or Word. Corrections must, however, be made as you go along. In contrast, the IBM system allows you to dictate whole paragraphs into a dictation window. Errors are corrected at the end before you transfer the text to the word processor of your choice. Both Dragon Dictate and IBM systems require the use of discrete speech, whereas the Phillips system allows you to dictate continuous speech. The Phillips system is optimised for supporting multiple users and secretaries over a network. The voice recognition is undertaken when the dictation has finished, and the system is designed for a secretary to listen to the dictation and make the corrections. In the future, speech recognition is likely to become a standard feature of operating systems.

# Desktop publishing

### Desktop publishing

- Ideal for handouts, patient information leaflets, etc
- Works like a paste board
- Much easier to control the precise position of figures and text than with a word processor
- Special effects such as drop caps, complex text flow around drawings, creative text art forms
- Advanced document management for large documents—page, figure, and chapter numbering; automatic indexing; cross referencing
- Wide range of import filters for text and graphics created in other programs
- Page grids for automatic alignment of text and graphics
- Colour separation and colour control for professional colour printing

If you plan to create a document containing a complex mixture of text, headings, subheadings, and graphics you should consider using desktop publishing. Laying out the page in a desktop publishing program is much easier because text and graphics are entered into individual boxes on the screen, which can then be moved around at will, allowing you to experiment with different layouts. The programs also contain templates for popular documents such as newsletters and brochures, which make designing a document even easier. There are now several excellent budget programs which offer more facilities than the average user is ever likely to need.

# Saving your work

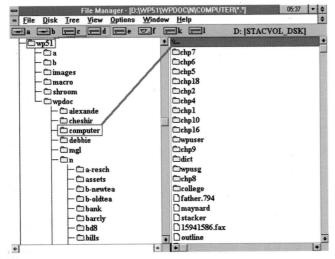

Organisation of files.

One of the advantages of word processors is that all your work can be saved on your hard disk or a floppy disk for later use. It is wise to save the document regularly as you type and to set the automatic save option of the program to "on" so that if you accidentally clear the screen or there is a power failure you will not lose the entire document.

Your computer's hard disk is essentially a filing cabinet. You should divide it into directories (drawers) with subdirectories (subdividers) so that you can easily find your filed material again. The word processor will suggest a main directory for storing your work, and it is a good idea to create subdirectories off this.

Most word processors require you to give your work a filename with a maximum of eight characters followed by a full stop and a three character extension—for example, document.jun. Some programs, however, allow longer, more informative filenames (Letter-to-John-Monday-5-June). It is a good idea to type the filename at the beginning of the document for later reference.

# Getting your thoughts on paper

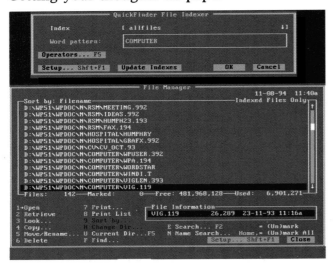

QuickFinder index for locating lost files

*Finding a file*

Even with detailed filenames and well organised subdirectories it can eventually become difficult to find a document again among the thousands on your computer. It helps to save a document summary with the file, but this requires some discipline.

A more efficient method is to use a text retrieval system such as that included in WordPerfect 6.0. The QuickFinder index can index every word in all the documents on the hard disk allowing instant searching of all words in your files.

## Useful names and telephone numbers

### Word processors

| | | |
|---|---|---|
| AmiPro | Lotus software's mainstream word processor | 01784 455445 |
| Claris Works | Well known to Macintosh users, now available for the PC | 0181 756 0101 |
| LetterPerfect | WordPerfect's budget word processor | 0800 177277 |
| PC Write | One of the best Shareware word processors | Shareware |
| Universal Word | A graphical word processor that handles foreign languages such as Arabic, Greek, etc | 01344 303800 |
| Word | Microsoft's flagship word processor | 01734 270000 |
| WordPerfect | The most popular word processor widely used in hospitals | 0800 973189 |
| Wordstar | An old favourite, now available for Windows | 0181 789 2000 |

### Utilities

| | | |
|---|---|---|
| Dragon Systems UK | Speech recognition system | 01242 678575 |
| Grammatik | Grammar checker | 0800 177277 |
| IBM VoiceType | Speech recognition system | 01329 242728 |
| Phillips Dictations Systems | Speech recognition system | 01206 755755 |
| Stedman's Medical Dictionary | Adds medical terminology to WordPerfect's dictionary. British and American versions available | 0171 385 2357 |
| Wordstar writing accessories | Correct letters, Correct quotes, Correct grammar, encyclopaedia | 0181 520 3502 |

### Desktop publishing

| | | |
|---|---|---|
| Microsoft Publisher | Probably the easiest to use budget program | 01734 270000 |
| Serif PagePlus | Fully featured budget program | 0800 924925 |
| Corel Ventura | Professional program | 0800 333333 |
| Adobe PageMaker | Professional program | 0181 606 4000 |
| WordPerfect User Group | Offers meetings, newsletter, help and advice for WordPerfect users | 01277 212545 |
| MS Word User Group | Similar help and advice for Word users | 01277 212545 |

# 6   STORING AND MANAGING DATA

Readers will be familiar with the traditional card index which is used to store relatively simple information such as a list of books in a library. Database programs are the electronic equivalent of a card index but offer several advantages. Most important of these is the ability to search and analyse the stored data rapidly and reliably. In addition to this, large amounts of information can be stored in a fraction of the space that would be required for equivalent paper records; several people on a network or multiuser system can use the same database simultaneously; and the results of searches can easily be printed in the form of a report. Furthermore, any stored data can be used by other programs such as a word processor (for creating circular letters or mailing labels), a spreadsheet (for manipulation and charting of the data), or a statistical program (for detailed analysis).

---

**Advantages of an electronic database**

Highly compact data storage
Fast and accurate searches
Easy to amend stored data
Easy data manipulation
Multiuser access
Printed reports
Ease of backup

---

## Structure of databases

Information stored in a database is broken down into manageable portions which are stored in separate compartments called fields and records. For example, a surname would be entered into one field, and the first name or initial and date of birth into subsequent fields. A collection of fields relating to one person or event is called a record. A database can contain an unlimited number of records.

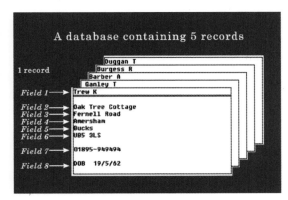

Simple flatfile database.

### Flatfile databases

Flatfile databases are the most basic type and are analogous to a card index. They are easy to create with any database program and are ideal for storing simple information such as a list of names and addresses. They offer all the facilities that many people are likely to need.

### Relational databases

In a relational database information is stored in several separate, cross referenced database files. Although more complex, this structure allows very powerful and efficient systems to be developed. A good example of this is a database containing basic information about a group of patients, including the name of the general practitioner with whom each patient is registered. In a flatfile database the name of the patient's general practitioner would have to be entered in every record. In a relational database you would enter the general practitioner's name just once into a separate small database. The patient's record is then designed to point to the correct doctor in the general practitioner database. The advantage of this approach is that the person entering patient data can be offered a list of general practitioners derived from the general practitioner database (called a pick list), which saves time and reduces the risk of error. Furthermore, if a doctor changes, it is necessary to alter only one record in the general practitioner database. The patients' records would then update automatically.

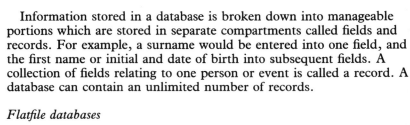

Patient Record

GP Database

Example of a relational database.

# Creating a database

## 1. Define the fields

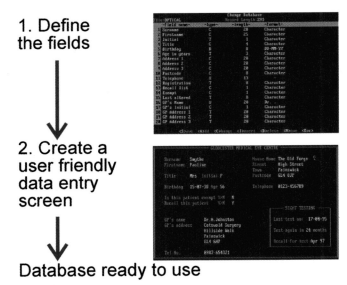

## 2. Create a user friendly data entry screen

## Database ready to use

Steps for creating a database.

Unlike with other programs such as word processors, which can be used immediately, you have to create the database structure before you can enter any data. Although designing flatfile databases is relatively straightforward and well within most people's capability, creating a relational database is more difficult.

Traditionally, it has been necessary to employ a professional programmer or to master a database programming language such as dBase. Handholding techniques such as Microsoft's Wizards have now made it easier to create quite complex databases without using a programming language. Nevertheless, unless you are already familiar with a database your time would probably be better spent explaining your needs to a programmer. It is very easy to invest considerable time and effort trying to write the program yourself but remain disappointed with the end result.

# Validation of data and error trapping

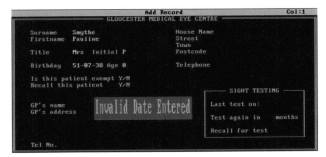

Some programs can be set up to detect errors automatically.

It is important to ensure that information is entered into the database consistently and accurately. Errors made during data entry often result in records being missed in a search. To reduce the possibility of error, many programs offer error trapping facilities that can be included in data entry screens. These could, for example, be used to define a valid age or height range so that bizarre mistakes such as men aged 164 years or women 4m tall are not accepted.

# Running the database

---

**Advantages of compiled databases**

Run faster
Can be distributed freely
No need for the main database program
Database structure cannot be inadvertently
   corrupted

---

The quality of reports is entirely dependent on the accuracy of the data entered.

**"Rubbish in, rubbish out"**

---

Once you have created and tested the database structure it can be run using the main database program. It is better, however, to use a compiling program to convert the database structure into a stand alone program. Alternatively use a "run-time" module, which is a small program capable of running your database without the need for the main program and which can usually be distributed freely to other users. Both of these methods prevent accidental damage to your database structure. Compiled databases have the additional advantage of running more quickly. Both techniques allow the database to be safely distributed to other users and are used by companies who market "ready to use" databases for specific purposes such as general practice systems.

To retrieve information from the database you need to search one or more fields. A simple search on a single field might, for example, be used to list all the patients with a particular surname or living in a given area. More complex searches of several fields using terms such as "and", "or", "if", and "not" could be used to identify a group such as all men aged under 60 who do not smoke but have coronary heart disease.

Most databases offer facilities to search for fragments of a name—for example, "Jo" could be used to search for Jones, Johnson, or Joseph. Other programs offer an option to expand the search to include similar sounding names spelt differently—for example, Smith and Smythe.

# Creating a report

**PATIENTS FOR RECALL**

RECALL MONTH: Nov 95   List Generated on:  17-09-95

| First Name | Surname | Address | Telephone |
|---|---|---|---|
| Sharon | Davies | Pilkington Court | 01452-504167 |
| Anne-Marie | Fellows | Rocking Road | 01452-615478 |
| John | Hartley | Riverside Close | 01452-619730 |
| Sandra | Lassiter | Sandhurst Lane | 01452-601875 |
| Mark | Leatham | Harrington Street | 01452-601815 |
| Safwabibi | Mustafa | 456 Falkner Street | 01452-951753 |
| Caroline | Peters | 52 Barlett Street | 01452-601508 |

**Total Number of Patients due for recall in Nov 95 = 7**

Recall list which can be used to generate a standard letter.

Gloucester Medical Eye Centre
London Road, Gloucester
Tel. 01452 - 381113

Mrs S Davies
Flat 3
Pilkington Court
Gloucester
GL1 4DR

17th September 1995

Dear Mrs Davies,

We note from our records that your last sight test was 12 months ago, and that your next test falls due very soon. It would help us greatly if you would ring as soon as possible to make an appointment in the first part of November.

The reception is open from 8.30am - 5.30pm Monday to Friday and from 8.30am - 1pm on Saturdays.

Yours sincerely,

Mrs J Sutherland
Secretary

Standard letter generated from recall list.

The results of a search can be used in several ways. You might, for example, want to view the results immediately on the screen, either one at a time or with all the results listed in a table. Alternatively, you could print the results in a report complete with subtotals and totals. Results can also be merged with a template to produce a personalised letter addressed to each person who meets the search criteria (as in call and recall systems). Once you have created a search strategy, it can be saved and used again as often as necessary.

Most databases allow you to export information in different file formats so that the data can be used by other programs. It is therefore important to ensure that the database is compatible with your chosen program.

## Database programs

**Flatfile databases:**

| | | |
|---|---|---|
| Cardbox-Plus | | 0171 470 7145 |
| Claris Filemaker Pro | | 0181 756 0101 |
| Button file (Shareware) | | 01297 552222 |
| File Express (Shareware) | | 01297 552222 |

**Relational databases**

| | | |
|---|---|---|
| Microsoft Access | Windows | 01734 270000 |
| Paradox | DOS and Windows | 0800 177277 |
| dBase | DOS and Windows | 01734 320022 |
| Superbase | Windows | 01344 867100 |
| Lotus Approach | Windows | 01784 445808 |
| Alpha Four | DOS and Windows | 01752 897100 |
| FoxPro | Windows | 01734 270000 |
| DataEase | DOS and Windows | 0181 554 0582 |

# 7 MANIPULATING AND ANALYSING DATA

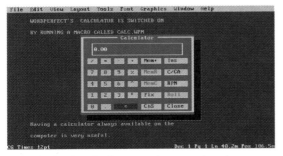

WordPerfect's calculator can be turned on by running the macro calc.wpm.

Spreadsheets form part of a family of tools for storing and manipulating numerical data. At their most basic, they perform the simple arithmetical calculations normally done on a handheld calculator. Several good programs are available that will simulate such calculators. Many of the calculator programs available provide facilities such as scientific functions, weight and measure conversions, and statistical and financial functions. They are often included in a package with other programs such as Windows or WordPerfect.

If you need to perform multiple calculations on a collection of data a spreadsheet program becomes invaluable. Spreadsheets were used before computers for bookkeeping and business accounts. However, maintaining accuracy when adding or performing the calculations on the figures within a spreadsheet was always a problem. A computer spreadsheet overcomes this problem. The calculations are always accurate, and if you make an alteration in a massive spreadsheet, the hundreds of calculations required to update the figures and totals are done in seconds.

## Structure of spreadsheets

|  | A | B | C |
|---|---|---|---|
| 1 |  | 120 |  |
| 2 |  | 145 |  |
| 3 |  | 156 |  |
| 4 |  | 223 |  |
| 5 |  | 195 |  |
| 6 |  | 135 |  |
| 7 |  | 198 |  |
| TOTAL |  | Sum(B1:B7) |  |
|  |  | 1172 |  |

The sum function is a quick way of adding up data in a spreadsheet.

A spreadsheet consists of columns labelled on the top A, B, C, D . . . and rows labelled on the left 1, 2, 3, 4. . . . The cells within the table are identified by the column and row label—for example, A1, A2, B1, B2. The column letter always goes first. You can enter numbers, formulas, or words into the cells. Entering a formula instructs the spreadsheet to carry out a calculation on data in other cells. For example, to add all the numbers in a column you would enter the formula B1 + B2 + B3 + B4 + B5 + B6 + B7 into the cell you wish the total to be placed or more simply use the summing function. If any of the numbers are altered the spreadsheet automatically recalculates the total.

The standard spreadsheet has available 9999 rows and 255 columns, making a total of over two million cells, all of which can be interlinked and used in mathematical calculations. This makes it a powerful tool that allows you to do complex analysis on small or large amounts of numerical data very rapidly.

## Functions

### Functions in spreadsheets

Arithmetical—Add, subtract, divide, multiply, sum, exponential, square root, count, log, power

Statistical—Row/column averages, maximum, minimum, standard deviations, median, random numbers

Trigonometrical—Pi, cos, sin, tan, acos, asin, atan

Calendar functions—Dates, time

Financial—currency, finance, term

Logical expressions—if, and, or, match, true, false, problem solving

Data sorting—Arranging in order text and numbers, distribution analysis

Spreadsheet programs all have several built in functions—that is, formulas that will automatically carry out calculations for which it would be time consuming to write the instructions in full each time using normal arithmetical symbols. They take the tedium out of long calculations and avoid the errors that inevitably occur when entering lengthy instructions. The big spreadsheets have over 300 of these functions available.

The date function is very useful as it allows dates or times to be used as numerical data. You can therefore automatically calculate a person's age from the date of birth. The problem solving function allows "what if?" questions to be asked. Here the problem solver tells you what values to use to make a particular formula equal to a value you specify.

# Sorting data

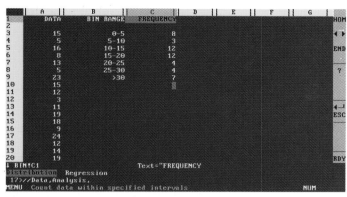

Spreadsheets will automatically sort your data to produce frequency distribution tables or charts.

Sorting data into ranges to create histograms or tables is laborious by hand. The advantage of storing data in a spreadsheet is that the program will create an accurate frequency distribution table, which can then be taken into a charting program or used by the charting functions of the spreadsheet program. Spreadsheets often have powerful charting capabilities which can also be incorporated into the spreadsheet itself to produce a professional looking report.

Spreadsheets are an excellent way of storing experimental or trial data. Each patient is allocated a separate row and each test result is then entered into the appropriate column, giving a clear representation of the data collected.

> **Advantages of computer spreadsheets over the paper equivalent**
>
> - Good overview of the data
> - Easy manipulation of the data
> - Able to print out a clear copy of the data
> - Transfer of data into and from other programs—for example, word processors, databases
> - Direct creation of charts for reports

Once the data have been entered into the spreadsheet it is easy to sort them into alphabetical or numerical order with the sorting function or perform complex calculations.

Many people prefer to use spreadsheets for small or moderate amounts of data rather than a database because of the complexities of setting up a database. However, for large amounts of data spreadsheets become unwieldy, and a database is much more suitable.

The data you have collected is invaluable so it is important to make regular back ups and keep a copy in a secure place away from work.

# Choosing a spreadsheet programme

| Patient | Age | Sex | Vision | | Refractive Error—Dioptres | |
|---|---|---|---|---|---|---|
| | | | Right | Left | Right | Left |
| 23 | 12 | F | †6/6 | 6/5 | −2·50 | −0·50 |
| 24 | 19 | M | †6/4 | 6/4 | −1·50 | −1·50 |
| 25 | 16 | M | †6/6 | 6/6 | +6·00/+0·75×90° | +6·50/+0·50×90° |
| 26 | 17 | M | †6/5 | 6/5 | −5·50 | −5·50/−0·75×90° |
| 27 | 8 mth | F | Not possible | | +9·00 | +10·00 |

A spreadsheet can be imported into a word processing program for presentation.

Three dimensional spreadsheet. Note the tabs at the bottom allowing you to switch between pages.

Many of the leading word processing packages contain quite powerful spreadsheets, though they are often referred to as tables. The advantages of using your word processor's spreadsheet are that you are working within a familiar program and you can produce a high quality looking document incorporating your spreadsheet. The formatting and printing abilities of some spreadsheet programs are more difficult to use than those of word processors and often not as good.

However, spreadsheets within a word processor, are not as easy to use to manipulate data as stand alone programs. If you work regularly with data you should use a proper spreadsheet program. To produce a high quality report you can import the spreadsheet into the word processing package or produce a direct link to your spreadsheet from the word processor. With a direct link the spreadsheet in your word processor will automatically be updated should you make any alterations in the spreadsheet.

## 3D spreadsheets

Modern spreadsheet programs allow you to load and view more than one spreadsheet at a time and to interlink the spreadsheets. For example, monthly financial data can be entered as a page for each month and then the whole linked as a single spreadsheet so that calculations can be performed between any cell

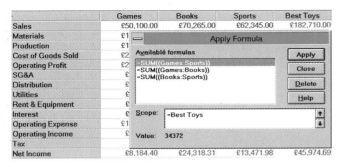

Some spreadsheets let you label the columns and rows with proper names.

Example of a multidimensional spreadsheet.

# Statistical analysis

Statistics programs are invaluable for research.

Arcus Pro-Stat offers comprehensive statistical guidance.

on any page. Many of these three dimensional spreadsheets allow you to label each spreadsheet page with a helpful name, and you can then use the mouse to click on the label or tab and bring up that spreadsheet page.

Manufacturers have tried hard to make spreadsheets more user friendly. One way they have done this is to allow labels such as column B to be replaced with more meaningful plain English terms such as "Games". To perform calculations you enter the names instead of abstract numbers and letters—for example Sum((Games:Sports)). Although this is long winded for simple spreadsheets, it greatly simplifies the use of multiple spreadsheets with complex arrangements of data.

*Multidimensional spreadsheets*

Spreadsheets have developed beyond three dimensions into multidimensional programs. This is not an easy concept to understand but considerably extends the capabilities of spreadsheets. In the figure the row numbers represent each entry and are the first dimension, the columns represent the description, amount, etc and are the second dimension, the expenses/income is the third, the month the fourth, the year the fifth, and the name of the account the sixth dimension.

In the example shown, by clicking with the mouse button on any of the dimensions it is possible to change the display to show, for example, the "Expenses" spreadsheet for the month of "January" in "1995" for "Mr Harvey's account". The display will show only two dimensions at once, but any combination of the dimensions can be applied to the x and y axes, resulting in a powerful analytical tool.

Statistical analyses are an integral part of most research projects. Until recently, statistical programs were both expensive and non-user friendly, but now many of the latest ones are menu driven and use the Windows or Macintosh graphic user interfaces. This has made the programs simpler to use, and budget packages will fit the pocket and needs of many people. Once you have entered the data into the program you simply select the correct statistical analysis from the menu and the calculations are done automatically.

The choice of statistical package will depend not only on your budget and experience but on the size and complexity of the analyses required. If you are doing a large study it is advisable to seek the advice of a statistician before starting the study to plan how the data will be collected and analysed. The planning stage should include a trial analysis of data with the proposed program.

Although these programs are not designed to replace the advice or work of a qualified statistician, they have a valuable role in allowing non-statisticians to analyse data without needing to use or understand fully the complex formulas behind them. All programs come with various levels of guidance on selecting the correct statistical analysis to use.

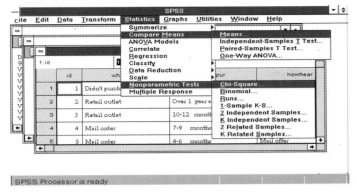

The SPSS package offers complex statistical programs.

Arcus, which is aimed at biomedical researchers in particular, has good on line help which is easy for beginners to understand yet is detailed enough to remain useful for experienced users. The heavyweight statistical packages like SPSS are supplied with several large manuals. These are fine for the statistician but too complex for the novice. Advanced programs also enable you to ask "what if?" questions—for example, which data values would be needed to reach statistical significance.

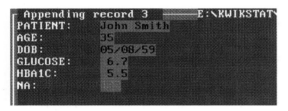

Some statistics programs offer database-like systems to minimise the number of keystrokes required to enter data.

### Entering and presenting data

One of the great benefits of computers is that you have to enter your data into a program only once. You can then usually transfer them to other programs. So, for instance, you could use a database to enter your data. This can make a lot of sense as the data entry mechanism is much more sophisticated and quicker than with a spreadsheet or a word processor. Thereafter you could transfer the data into a spreadsheet, into a statistics program for analysis, and finally into a word processor for printing the final report.

Some of the statistics programs have data entry facilities that are like those of a database. Once you have entered the number or name the cursor will either automatically move on to the next entry box or may be moved by pressing the return key. Many statistics programs can also create charts directly from your data and offer some of the specialist plots that are not routinely found on the standard business charting programs.

## Sources of programs for manipulating data

**Calculators:**

| | | |
|---|---|---|
| Microsoft Windows | Basic and scientific calculator included in the standard Windows program | 01734 270000 |
| Calc Plus | DOS based "reverse Polish logic" calculator. Also wide range of other calculators available as Shareware | 01892 663298 |
| WordPerfect | Activated by running the macro Calc.wpm in WP5.1 or WP6.0 | 0800 973189 |

**Spreadsheets:**

| | | |
|---|---|---|
| Quattro Pro | Fully featured three dimensional with notebook style indexing | 0800 177277 |
| Lotus 1-2-3 | Very well known three dimensional and multidimensional spreadsheet with versions for DOS, Windows, and O/S2 | 01784 455445 |
| CA-Supercal | Range of spreadsheets from three dimensional DOS applications to windows multidimensional spreadsheet | 01753 679679 |
| Microsoft Excel | Fully featured 3D with notebook style indexing | 01734 270000 |

**Statistical Programmes:**

| | | |
|---|---|---|
| Arcus Pro-Stat | Written for doctors. DOS and Windows version. Contains all useful statistical functions in a user friendly environment. Windows based | 01695 424034 |
| C-Stat | Originates from the Radcliffe Infirmary Oxford. DOS and Windows based | 01865 784800 |
| EpiInfo | Can be downloaded free from the Internet (http://www.crawford.com/epo/epi/epi.html) | |
| Kwikstat | Shareware based program very popular in United States | 001214 291 2115 |
| Minitab | Comprehensive program available for DOS, Windows, Macintosh, Unix | 01203 695730 |
| Nanostat | Simple to use and can run on a minimum specification computer; available in French and Italian | 0171 833 3056 |
| SAS | Large general purpose program popular in the pharmaceutical industry | 01628 486933 |
| SPSS-PC+ | Practically nothing it can't do but expensive | 01932 566262 |
| STATA | Medically oriented DOS, Windows, and Macintosh | 0181 462 0093 |
| StatSoft | Comprehensive statistical program with integrated graphics | 01462 482822 |
| Statgraphics | Very powerful and well known for its integrated graphics | 0171 436 9481 |
| SYSTAT | General statistic package | 0181 462 0093 |
| UNISTAT | Wide range of statistical analysis and charting capabilities | 0181 964 1130 |

# 8 ILLUSTRATING AND PRESENTING DATA

## Text Slide

- Template ensures consistent style
- Easy to enter text and see style
- Save your own style
- Can use for slides or overhead projections
- Slide shows with computer projections

Simple text slide created with a word processor.

Good quality slides, overheads, and handouts are essential when giving a presentation whether it is a seminar, lecture, or paper at a scientific meeting. They provide a reassuring framework for your talk, help maintain the audience's interest, and make sure the salient points are remembered.

## Text based illustrations

Displaying your key points is a powerful way of focusing the mind of the audience. Text slides or overheads are one of the most useful types of illustrations to create and form the basis of most presentations. The most basic method for making them is to use a word processor attached to an inkjet or laser printer which can print on to acetate sheets for overhead projection or on to paper for the photographic department to make into a slide. Laser quality thermal acetates can be put through most printers or photocopiers.

The more advanced word processors allow considerable embellishment to the presentation. And if you have a colour printer, it is just as easy to produce colour overheads–even on the night before the presentation.

*Liquid crystal display panels*

Liquid crystal display (LCD) colour panels link directly to the computer, allowing the computer image to be projected on to a large screen. This avoids the need for acetate sheets. Most presentation packages include a slide show facility, which allows your slides to be displayed one after the other. Producing the presentation is cheap, but the cost of the additional equipment is high. The system is therefore more appropriate for permanent lecture facilities.

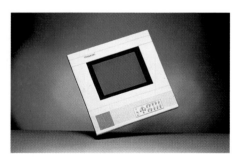

Liquid crystal display panel.

## Making slides

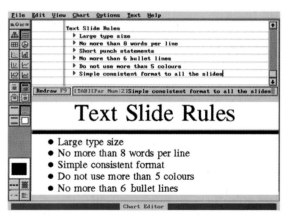

Software packages have made making slides easier.

Creating 35 mm slides is as easy as making overhead sheets but often requires a little more time to make up the slides. Modern desktop computers and presentation software allow you to do all the preparatory work yourself. This has the advantage of giving you total control of the design. The illustrations can then be sent on disk to the medical illustration department or a bureau to produce the photographic slides.

It is best to use a presentation software package to create slides. These packages are designed to create eye catching charts simply and quickly. The commonest mistake is to put too much information on the slide and confuse the audience. Adopt a consistent style for the format and colour scheme for your slides. All programs include templates, which greatly simplify the process of creating a presentation.

Many packages use an outline format. The outline displays the plain text without the colour or font size added, and the result is displayed at the same time in the lower half of the frame. Any changes can quickly be seen. The style of the text or bullets is changed from the pull down menus. Once you have set your template and saved it you can recall it later to create another presentation. Though the outline method may seem unfamiliar at first, it allows you to enter text rapidly. There are four basic methods of producing slides:

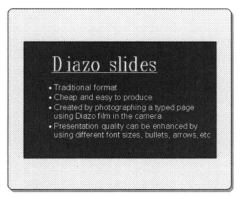

Diazo slides are quick and cheap.

*Diazo slides*

Although diazo slides are traditionally produced with a typewriter, the quality can be greatly enhanced by creating the original with an advanced word processor or a presentation package. Larger fonts, borders, and bullets all increase the impact.

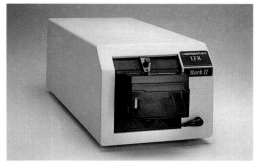

Negative slides are cheap and easy to produce.

*Negative slides*

These are produced by printing the presentation on to paper and then photographing it using a black and white negative film. The white text on a black background gives impact, but as the background colour is black the auditorium can seem very dark.

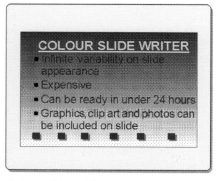

Colour slide writing machines are expensive but give good results.

*Colour slides*

This slightly more expensive format is very useful when combining printed colour pictures (such as a photograph) with some additional text. The text can be printed on to A4 paper, any pictures pasted on to it, and the whole sheet photographed. The white background of the final slide proves a light and pleasing slide format.

*Slide writer*

Colour slide writing machines produce stunning high quality slides straight from the computer. These machines are expensive and so are usually found only in medical illustration departments. Alternatively, numerous bureaus will accept your work either by post on a floppy disk or by modem for a rapid service. It is best to use the same software package as that used by the photographic department or bureau to avoid problems with file compatibility.

Colour slide writing machine.

# Charts

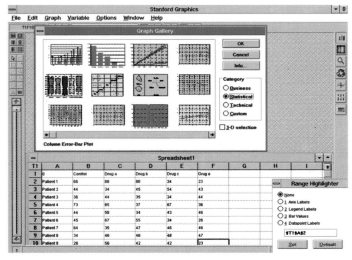

Package for making data into a chart.

Charts convey a message more effectively than numbers in a table. The leading presentation software packages offer about 200 types of chart. Data are entered in a similar way to those for a spreadsheet and can be imported from other programs. Once the data are entered they are easy to manipulate. Many programs work in colour, but you will often need only black and white.

Organisational charts are useful to illustrate staffing arrangements of departments, family trees, or algorithms. General charting programs often include basic organisational charts, but a dedicated organisational charting program is more flexible.

# Drawing and graphics packages

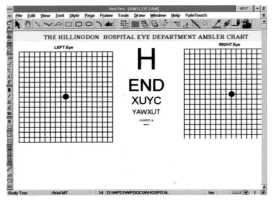

Simple drawing package with a word processor.

Illustrations can convey a great deal of information very quickly. Few of us are natural artists, but with the aid of computer drawing software, scanned images, and a bundle of clip art most people can produce acceptable drawings. This requires a little practice, and it is best to start by running through the tutorial that comes with the software and then trying something simple.

These vector drawing programs all offer several basic tools such as simple shapes (squares, circles, triangles, polygons) and lines (straight, curved, polylines, and arrows). The shapes can be connected and filled with patterns or colour. The number of drawing tools and the ability to alter the line types and fill of an object varies among packages.

Most large word processing packages include simple drawing tools which are sufficient for basic pictures and can also annotate scanned images.

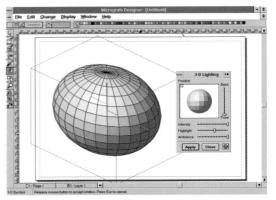

Clip art from a graphics package.

### Graphics packages

The budget graphic programs have an extensive range of drawing capabilities that will be more than adequate for the average user. They run quickly on even a modest machine. The leading drawing packages such as Corel Draw and Micrografx Designer include over 13 000 clip art images on CD ROM and more than 200 different fonts. The packages are easy to use and capable of handling the most complex tasks, but they do require a powerful computer.

### Three dimensional drawing

The more powerful programs allow you to work in three dimensions. This is done by either extruding a two dimensional image or using three dimensional building blocks to create the drawing. Manipulation in three dimensions is easily done around the x, y, and z axes.

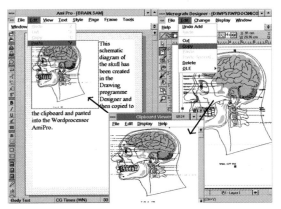

Graphics packages let you work in three dimensions.

### Clip art

You may be able to find a suitable ready made drawing from the clip art supplied with your drawing or presentation packages. There is a wealth of commercial clip art available both on floppy disk and on CD ROM.

### Photo CD

When developing ordinary 35 mm photographic slides or negatives you can get the photographs copied on to a CD ROM. If your computer has Photo CD compatible software you can then import pictures taken with your camera into your work.

# Transferring data

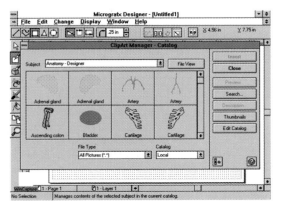

Transferring data across two Windows programs.

Transferring graphic images between different programs can cause problems because there are over 23 different file formats, but most major programs offer a range of export and import facilities. Transfer is easiest within Windows–the image is simply copied to the clipboard and then pasted into the other program.

# Scanners

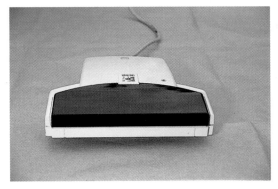

Handheld scanner.

Scanners greatly increase the scope for producing presentations and handouts. They allow images to be transferred from the printed page to a computer and then incorporated into the working document. There are two basic types.

### Handheld scanners

A handheld scanner is the cheapest. It is moved across the stationary paper and is particularly suitable for small images. Larger images can be scanned in 10 cm widths that are then stitched together by the software. Line diagrams or logos are scanned in as line art, with the image made up of only black and white pixels. This format takes the least memory but is not suitable for photographs, which need grey scale imaging. Here each pixel may be represented by a shade of grey with up to 8, 16, or 256 shades depending on the resolution set. Line art generally prints very well from a standard laser or ink jet printer, but the quality of grey scale images varies between printers.

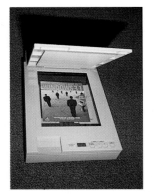

Flatbed scanner.

### Flatbed scanner

A beam of light passes across the stationary paper, similar to a photocopier. These scanners are ideal for A4 size images and give better resolution than a hand scanner. Colour scanners are more expensive, and you should remember that an A4 size image scanned at 600 dots per inch in 24 bit colour will occupy a massive 11 megabytes of disk space. You will therefore need to have a fast processor and lots of memory (RAM). By keeping images small, however, it is possible to manipulate colour pictures on a powerful computer. Colour images are particularly suitable if you are going to use a slide writer or colour printer for the final output.

A flatbed scanner with optical character recognition software can also scan in passages of text. The text is scanned as ASCII characters that can then be incorporated into a word processor. Scanners do, however, produce a lot of inaccuracies, which makes scanning large documents difficult.

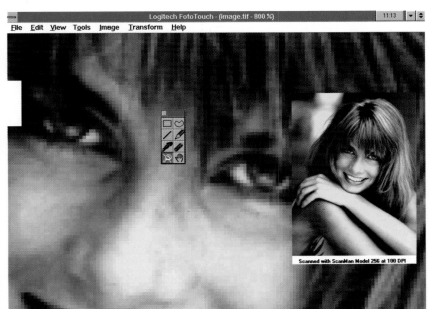

Scanned images can be edited to improve their appearance.

### Editing scanned images

Scanned images are stored as bit mapped images. They are made up of pixels and can be edited rather like a painting with brush-like tools and erasers. This allows you to remove unwanted material and to touch up and add to the image. With grey scale images you can alter the contrast, brightness, and tone. Once you have finished editing the image can be copied into the document or slide.

## Useful names and telephone numbers

**Drawing programs**

| | | |
|---|---|---|
| Arts and Letters | Excellent collection of cartoon style graphics | 001 214 661 8960 |
| Corel Draw | Leading drawing suite of programs with CD ROM | 0800 333333 |
| CA-Cricket Paint | Easy to use program for adjusting scanned and bit mapped images | 01753 577733 |
| Micrografx Designer | Professional technical drawing with CD ROM | 0800 626009 |
| Micrografx Graphics Works | Excellent budget package with CD ROM | 0800 626009 |
| Professional Draw | Flexible budget drawing package | 01753 832383 |
| Top Draw | Shareware object oriented drawing package | 01442 891331 |
| Visio | Organisational charting and drag and drop drawing | 0800 834859 |
| ChemWindow | Designed for drawing and managing chemical structures | 01865 784800 |

**Presentation and charting programs**

| | | |
|---|---|---|
| Freelance Graphics | Lotus's top range program aimed at presentations | 01784 455445 |
| Harvard Graphics | Well known charting program | 01344 867100 |
| Microsoft PowerPoint | Leading program for presentation | 01734 270000 |
| Standford Graphics | Scientific charting program with statistical analysis | 01462 480055 |
| WordPerfect Presentations | Integrates with WordPerfect available for DOS and Windows | 0800 973189 |

**Equipment**

| | | |
|---|---|---|
| Logitech Scanners | Handheld scanners | 01344 891313 |
| Epson | Flatbed scanners | 01442 61144 |
| Lasergraphics LFR | Slide makers | 01753 830999 |

# 9 LINKING YOUR COMPUTER TO THE OUTSIDE WORLD

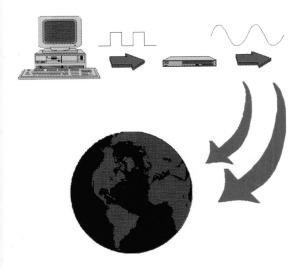

The international telephone network has over 400 million subscribers This vast network can be used to connect even the most basic personal computer to any other computer or information system anywhere in the world. Most of these systems are available 24 hours a day, seven days a week, and can be accessed very easily from home or work using simple and cheap equipment. This means anyone can tap into the world's accumulated medical knowledge at the touch of a button.

Computers communicate internally by digital signals. Although these signals can be sent down a wire, the telephone network has been designed to carry speech-like frequencies. For computers to use telephone lines their digital signals have to be converted to speech frequencies. This conversion is carried out by a modem (modulator-demodulator).

## Selecting a modem

---

### What you need to link up to other computers

*Computer*—Virtually any computer, provided it has a serial port

*Modem:*
External—Mains powered unit with a speaker and visual display unit to show status of modem
Internal—Slots directly into an expansion socket inside the computer
Pocket—Battery powered portable unit ideal for notebooks
PCMCIA—Credit card sized internal modem for notebooks

*Telephone line*—Good quality lines improve reliability of connection

*Communication software*—The interface between computer and modem making it easy to operate

*Password*—Permission is usually required to gain access to another computer

---

There are several points to consider when buying a modem. Most countries allow only approved modems to be connected to their public telephone network. The stamp of approval guarantees compatibility. Because the standards vary, manufacturers have to produce a specific modem for each country, although a pan-European standard is being discussed. It is no longer worth buying a modem that cannot also send faxes.

Configuring your communications program to match a given modem can sometimes be difficult, but it is much easier if the modem you purchase is directly supported by the software. The quality and ease of access of technical support varies, and good support from a British or locally based company is of great help when problems arise. The performance of modems varies considerably depending on two main factors: the basic speed of the modem (quoted as the Baud rate) and data compression.

---

### CCITT communication standards (Communication Comité Consultatif Internationale de Télégraphique Téléphonique)

| Standards | Baud rate | Transfer time of 100 kb file |
|-----------|-----------|------------------------------|
| V21 | 300 | 56 min |
| V23 | 1200/75 | 14 min |
| V22bis | 2400 | 7 min |
| V32 | 9600 | 1 min 42 s |
| V32bis | 14 400 | 1 min 12 s |
| V34 and VFast | 28 800 | 34 s |

---

*Speed or Baud rate*

The Baud rate is an indication of the speed at which data can be exchanged, a higher number equating to faster transfer. At 2400 Baud a 100 kb file containing 50 pages of A4 text or 75 references will take about seven minutes to transfer; at 28 800 Baud this is reduced to 34 seconds. If you regularly access a database with high online charges over a long distance telephone line or if you plan to transfer very large volumes of data, consider buying a faster modem. The newest modems offer superb performance, but leading edge technology is always more expensive. Most users will find that a slightly slower modem will satisfy their needs and offer better value for money.

# Linking your computer to the outside world

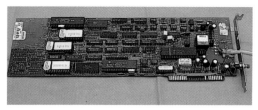

Internal card modem.

### Error correction and data compression packages

*Microcom Network Protocols (MNP)*
Class 1—Very basic error correction. Data are sent in only one direction at a time
Class 2—Data can be sent in both directions
Class 3—Synchronous data transfer
Class 4—Data phase optimisation further improves transfer speed
Class 5—Data compression added with up to ×2 speed increase

*Comité Consultatif Internationale de Télégraphique Téléphonique (CCITT)*
V42—Sophisticated error correction
V42bis—Dynamic data compression added with up to ×4 speed increase

*Error correction and data compression*

The quality of telephone lines has improved enormously, but noise does sometimes occur. This will corrupt the data being transferred, and it is therefore essential that both modems have an automatic error correcting capability. There are two main standards, although MNP (Microcom Network Protocol) has now been largely superseded by the more advanced and robust CCITT (Comité Consultatif Internationale de Télégraphique Téléphonique) V42 protocol.

To improve the data throughput further modems compress the data being transferred. MNP class 5 allows data to be transferred at up to twice the normal rate. Again this has largely been superseded by the more advanced CCITT V42bis protocol, which increases the data transfer rate by a factor of up to four. In addition V42bis can analyse the type of data being transferred and dynamically optimise the degree of data compression. Most modern modems can use both V42 error correction and V42bis data compression.

Once you have bought your modem and set up the software, there is no need to worry about the various standards because whenever two modems establish a connection (handshake) they automatically negotiate the best protocol to use.

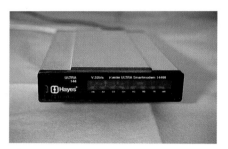

External modem with mains power supply.

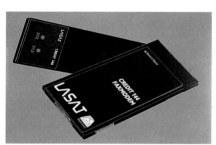

PCMCIA (PC card) modem.

## Selecting communications software

### Communications software

*Commercial*
HyperTerminal is included in Windows 95
Hayes Smartcom DOS/Windows (01252 775500)
Procom plus DOS/Windows
Crosstalk DOS/Windows

*Shareware*
Odyssey DOS/Windows
Telix DOS/Windows

*Apple*
Vicom (01202 293233)

*Fax software*
Delrina Winfa/Dosfax (0181 207 3163)

*Online services*
BMA Library—Symantex PC Anywhere (01703 638868)
CompuServe—CompuServe Information Manager DOS/Windows
Internet—See next chapter

Many communication programs are available and all have similar basic capabilities. Shareware libraries such as Software Source (01297 552222) offer several excellent low cost programs which you can legally try before you buy. However, access to some databases (for example, BMA Medline) is enhanced by more powerful software.

Some information services (for example, CompuServe (0800 289458) and BT's Phone Base (0800 919199)) have their own dedicated software, which makes them easier to use.

Previously many people used DOS rather than Windows communications software because communication was faster and more reliable under DOS. However, Windows 95 includes an excellent communications program called HyperTerminal. For many users, this is all that will be needed to connect to a wide variety of places. Furthermore, Windows 95 allows you to create an icon on your desktop for services such as BMA Medline. Double clicking on this icon launches HyperTerminal and automatically connects you to the service.

# Setting up the software

## Setup procedures

*Communication port*—The software needs to know which communication (COM) port the modem is connected to. Usually COM1 or COM2

*Modem type*—Modern software greatly simplifies the setup by allowing you to select the name of the modem from an internal list

*Speed*—Normally set to the Baud rate of your modem but should be increased if data compression is used

*Terminal type*—The communications software can make your computer emulate many different types of terminal. Most online services will tell you which terminal type to select

*Passwords/scripts*—This greatly speeds logging on and avoids the need to remember various passwords

*Hardware test*—Software programmes like pcAnywhere allow a diagnostic test to ensure setup is complete

Before accessing another computer for the first time you need to contact the system operator (Sysop) to obtain a user guide and password. Remembering a different password for each service can be difficult. To solve this problem most good communications programs can record and replay the log on procedure. The recording is saved in a script file. Choosing the correct software setting for each service can seem daunting, but most user guides contain clear instructions on how to do this. These settings can then be saved under the name of the service for future use.

# Making the connection

## Direct dial and network services

*Direct dial services*
BMA Medline service
Phone Base
Bulletin boards

*National networks*
British Telecom—PSS and DialPlus Service
CompuServe
Data Star services
Internet
ISTEL Infotrack
JANET (joint academic network)

Though some services allow you to dial direct, others can only be accessed through a network. In some cases dialling into a network has the advantage that it can be accessed close to your home or office, thus saving you the cost of a long distance phone call. Contact individual services for details. The cost of using online database and networks varies considerably. Some are quite expensive whereas others are free.

Ordinary phone lines are analogue and it takes 15 seconds or more to make a connection. An alternative is a digital line or ISDN line (Integrated Service Digital Network), which will make the connection in under a second and transmit at 64 000 Baud. It is ideal for larger organisations with multiple sites or for video conferencing.

# Computer security and viruses

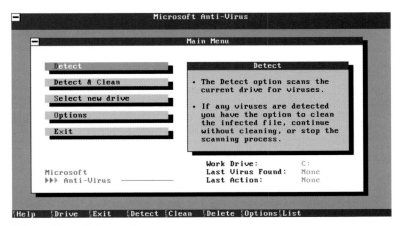

Microsoft's antivirus software.

Once your computer is connected to the telephone system, it is theoretically possible that someone may make unauthorised access to your system or that a computer virus will be transferred. However, by default modems can answer the telephone only if you instruct them to do so, and this protects the computer from attempts to gain unauthorised access.

Viruses cannot be acquired by merely accessing another computer, performing a search, and transferring text files. Computer viruses attach themselves to programs. Therefore, if programs are transferred there is a small risk that they may contain a virus. Most reputable operators go to extensive lengths to ensure their system is virus free, and contrary to popular belief the spread of viruses in this way is rare. Nevertheless, you should check all such programs with a virus scanner before using them.

# Obtaining help on computer related problems

## Sources of help

Telephone help lines
Manufacturers' online bulletin boards
Online forums
Information centres
Faxes and fax back services
Writing a letter

Modern computers and software are immensely complex and you will inevitably encounter problems. With the modem you can get support on CompuServe, CIX (Computer Information Exchange (0181 296-9666)), or the Internet. You post your question on to an electronic notice board for all to read. This will often result in helpful replies from more experienced users. These large message areas are also supported by the manufacturers, enabling you to communicate directly with the programmers. Alternatively, you can send a message by email or by fax to the manufacturers. As a last resort you can always write a letter. With this amount of help and support available no computer user should ever feel isolated.

## Other computerised services available via a modem

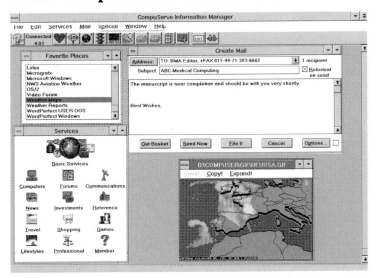

CompuServe provides a wide range of online services as well as access to the Internet.

A wide range of other services are available via your modem. For example, you can dial directly into BT's Phone Base, from which you can obtain not only the telephone number but also the full postal address for the price of a short phone call. Sending a fax is quicker and often cheaper than sending a letter and you get an acknowledgment of receipt. Any document created by your computer can be sent directly to its destination through a fax modem saving the trouble of printing it out first. Alternatively it can be sent via a fax server run by organisations such as CompuServe or BT's Mail Box.

Though sending a fax from a computer is easy, receiving is less convenient. If you have a fax modem then the computer has to be left on with the fax software running in a standby mode. This is often not practical, and stand alone fax machines remain the most convenient way to receive faxes.

## Computerised medical information services

### Online databases

**General medical:**
BIOSIS Previews—Database covering the entire field of life sciences; 9000 journals are indexed as well as monographs, reports, and symposia
Excerpta Medica[1 2 5 8]—Biomedical database especially strong on European journals and pharmacology. Covers 3500 journals, proceedings, books, and dissertations
Medline[1 2 4 5]—Major database of clinical medicine, indexing over 3700 journals with full abstracts
Science Citation Index[5 8]—Indexing over 7000 journals including article's list of references

**Specialised databases:**
Aids Database[1 2]—Bibliographic database with independent abstracts from the Bureau of Hygiene and Tropical Disease, London
BMA Press Cuttings[1 2]—Database of press cuttings on current medical affairs (updated daily)
Cancerlit[1 2]—Oncology citations and abstracts
Forensic Science[2]—Wide range of material related to forensic casework
General Practitioner[2]—Full text articles relating to business side of general practitioners' work
HSELINE[1]—United Kingdom Health and Safety Executive. Information covering all areas of health and safety at work
Inside information[5 8]—A million articles added each year from 10 000 most popular titles of the British lending library
Lancet[2]—Full text of the articles can be retrieved
Nursing and Allied Health[1 2]—Bibliographic index to most English language nursing journals

**Books or proceedings databases:**
Blaise-Line[5 6 7]—British Library's national bibliographic service with a comprehensive index of both books in and out of print
Index to Scientific and Technical Proceedings[5 8]—Information on the published proceedings of 4200 conferences a year

**Pharmacology**
International Pharmaceutical Abstracts[1 2]—Comprehensive coverage of worldwide pharmaceutical literature
Toxbase[3]—United Kingdom Poisons Information Service database
Travax[3]—Continually updated information on immunisations, malaria prevention, and other infection hazards for travellers abroad
Vadis[3]—Viewdata Drug Information Service offering additional information to that available in the *British National Formulary, Monthly Index of Medical Specialities,* and *Data Sheet Compendium*

The range of online information services is huge and continuing to grow. If you have a problem the chances are there is someone, somewhere who will be able to help you. The main difficulty is knowing what services are available and where to look. For instance there are over 3000 online databases currently listed, of which many are related to medicine.

The most popular medical database is Medline, which indexes over 3700 medical journals. It consists of over 8 million articles dating from 1966, 75% of which contain an abstract. Though there are several ways of accessing Medline, the best option for BMA members is to use the BMA library's online search facility. This service is free to members. Medline does not include reports, published proceedings of meetings, books, or work published before 1966. The four general medical databases each have a different emphasis with only about a 37% overlap. To do a complete search on a topic you will therefore need to access other databases. Of particular note is the science citation index, which indexes not only the articles but also the references. Searching the references in these articles locates older publications that predate electronic indexing. There are also numerous specialised databases which concentrate on providing an in depth index to all types of work in one specialty.

To help you decide where to search there are databases such as the Cross Database (via Data Star) which combine the indexes from many other sources. Searching this global index will indicate which of the databases is likely to contain the information you require.

Telephone numbers to ring for further information:
1 Data Star Services and Dialog 0171 930 5503
2 CompuServe Information Services 0800 289458
3 NHS Viewdata Information Services 0131 536 2298
4 BMA Library 0171 383 6184
5 JANET (Joint Academic Network) 01235 822212
6 Internet (for example, Unipalm Pipex 01223 250120)
7 National Bibliographic Service 01937 546585
8 Bath Information and Data Service 01225 826074

# 10   THE INTERNET

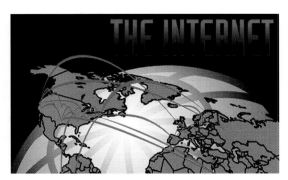

The Internet is a huge network of computers that spans the globe. It originated in the late 1960s from an American military project which was intended to provide reliable communications in the event of a nuclear war. The network started with just four computers but grew rapidly over the next few years. An estimated 40 million computers are now connected to it, and this number is growing by about 10% each year. Although access was originally restricted to government departments and organisations such as universities, the Internet has recently been opened up to everybody. It is now used by people and organisations from all walks of life including commercial organisations, university departments, hospitals, and medical schools, as well as a growing number of individual users dialling in from home.

## What does it do?

| Services available on the Internet |
| --- |
| • Information browsing |
|    Commercial |
|    Non-commercial |
| • Electronic mail (email) |
| • File transfer |
| • Newsgroups |

The Internet is best regarded as a framework which allows the free exchange of information between computers. With new services and users connecting to the network every day, it is becoming increasingly valuable as an information resource and communications superhighway. Among other things, it is now possible to access thousands of databases at universities and other research centres all over the world, read electronic journals, view and buy products from numerous companies, exchange news and views on a wide range of specialist subjects, and send virtually instantaneous electronic mail to any organisation, company, or individual connected to the Internet.

## How do I get on to the Internet?

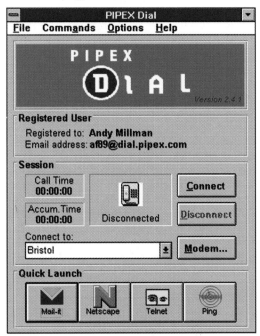

An integrated internet access package.

Accessing the Internet is very easy. You need a computer and a modem connected to a telephone line, and you will also need to contact an Internet service provider who will supply you with suitable software to load on to your computer, an Internet telephone number and password, an email address, and access to a help desk. Good software will store the telephone number of your service provider and your password during installation, and after that clicking on the connect button will automatically log you on to the net within a few seconds.

When selecting a service provider you should consider not only the initial connection charge and monthly service costs, but also the distance to the nearest access point. You may be able to find a local service provider but, if not, several of the larger companies offer a range of access points (called virtual points of presence or POPs) all over the country. Long distance telephone calls add considerably to the cost of using the service. One of the greatest advantages of the Internet is that connection to any other computer, whether it is just down the road or on the other side of the world, should cost no more than a local phone call.

## What to do when connected

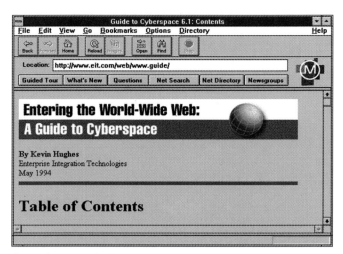

Accessing a typical worldwide web page with the Netscape browser.

Once you have connected to the Internet you normally see the service provider's home page, which is a like a menu. The page gives information about how to use and get the most from the Internet. It will also guide you towards search facilities which scan the Internet for the information or products that you require and FTP (file transfer protocol) sites which store programs, pictures, sound, and video files that you can download for use on your own computer.

The worldwide web (often referred to as WWW) is the most recent and interesting development on the Internet. It offers user friendly access to millions of pages of information on computers all over the world. To access the web you need a graphical browsing program (running under Windows, Macintosh, or OS/2). A program such as Netscape or Mosaic should be supplied as part of the package you purchase from the Internet service provider. The Windows 95 plus pack contains a new browser called Explorer.

## Navigating the worldwide web

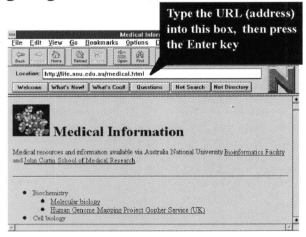

Hypertext links are the easiest way to navigate the worldwide web.

Almost every page on the web has a number of hypertext links to other pages on the same computer or to pages stored on another computer (often on the other side of the world). These appear as coloured text and are the easiest way to navigate around the Internet. Simply clicking on the text with the mouse takes you to the relevant page within a few seconds. Browsing programs keep a temporary list of the pages that you have viewed during a session, and it is easy to move backwards or forwards through the list one page at a time. You can also get a pull down list of the pages that have been accessed and go directly to any given page. Particularly useful pages can be tagged with a permanent bookmark, which allows you to return to that page at any time in the future.

### Useful worldwide web addresses

| Description | Location address (URL) |
| --- | --- |
| Yahoo | http://www.yahoo.com |
| BMJ | http://www.bmj.com/bmj |
| The virtual hospital | http://indy.radiology.uiowa.edu/VirtualHospital.html |
| Visible human project | http://www.nlm.nih.gov/extramural_research.dir/visible_human.html |
| World Health Organisation | http://www.who.ch |
| Professional Medicare | http://gnn.com/wic/wics/med.promed.html |
| GP-UK Homepage | http://www.ncl.ac.uk/~nphcare/GPUK/gpukhome.html |
| Primary Health Care Specialist Group | http://www.ncl.ac.uk/~nphcare/PHCSG//homepage.html |
| Jump—Selected points of entry to the web | http://www.ic.ac.uk/ccs/nss/jump.html |
| HealthNet | http://debra.dgbt.doc.ca/~mike/healthnet |
| Interactive Yellow Pages | http://netcenter.com/lite/cgi-bin/yellowsindex.pl |

*Uniform resource locator (URL)*

All web sites have an Internet address termed a uniform resource locator (URL). If you know the address for a particular web site, type it into the location box of your browser and you will automatically be connected to the correct site. The box gives some useful addresses that you could use as a starting point for exploring the Internet using hypertext links and bookmarks. You should, however, bear in mind that the Internet is constantly evolving and that addresses do change sometimes. Up to date lists of addresses can be found in Internet magazines and increasingly in medical journals.

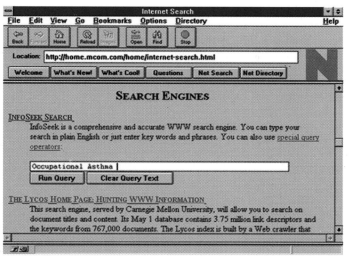

Search engines will help you find what you need.

*Searching for information*

Because the Internet is so large it is important to have an efficient way of finding the information that you need. Fortunately, there are now several computers dedicated to indexing the information scattered all over the world. These computers can easily be searched for any word or phrase, university, company, or subject.

Popular search engines include InfoSeek (http://www.infoseek.com/home) or Lycos (http://lycos.cs.cmu.edu). These services offer the casual user a limited number of hits free of charge, but comprehensive results are available only to subscribers. Alternatively, you can use Yahoo (http://www.yahoo.com), which displays information in the form of a tree, has extensive records of health care resources, and is entirely free. All the search systems present results in hypertext format. It is therefore very simple to browse through the search results to find exactly what you want.

# Electronic mail

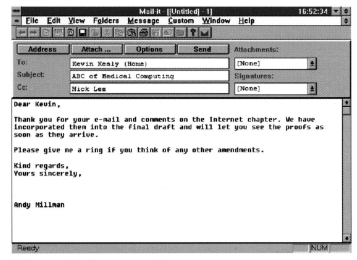

Using email software to send a message.

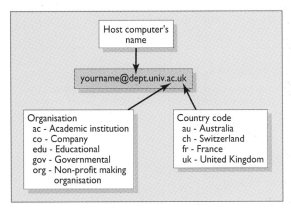

How an email address is derived.

Email ranks alongside the worldwide web as one of the main attractions of the Internet. It allows you to send messages to other people in just a few seconds even if they are thousands of miles away. You pay only the cost of the telephone call to your service provider. The same message can just as easily be broadcast to a group of people. In addition to simple text, you can send documents, graphics, sound files, and even programs, although you will need additional software (UU encoding/decoding) to do this. You could, for example, send a note to a colleague asking for an opinion on a clinical photograph, research data in a spreadsheet, or even a set of slides for a lecture.

Although you can write messages while connected to the Internet, it is more cost effective to write your messages before connection (off line). Your service provider will usually supply you with a program to do this. The program puts all your outgoing mail into a packet which is automatically dispatched the next time you dial into the Internet, while messages addressed to you are simultaneously delivered to your computer.

It is not uncommon to get a reply to an email message within a few minutes. If an email message cannot be delivered for any reason (for example, an incorrect email address) the system will usually let you know, but there is no reliable way of telling if someone has not dialled in to collect the message.

## The Internet

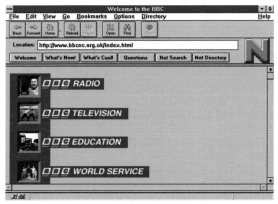

The BBC's web pages provide a wealth of information about its programmes.

### Commercial services

Companies and organisations are increasingly realising that the Internet offers an unrivalled opportunity to reach a global market. In most cases they offer information on and support for their products, but some are now offering items or services for sale. For example, you can look up flight information, book an airline ticket, and arrange hire car and hotel accommodation at any time of the day from the comfort of your own home. Secure systems which allow you to pay for these goods and services by credit card are being developed, but if they are not available it is best not to send credit card numbers across the net in case of interception. Some secure systems can be recognised by the use of https:// at the beginning of the address, or your browser may display a helpful icon such as a key.

## Transferring files

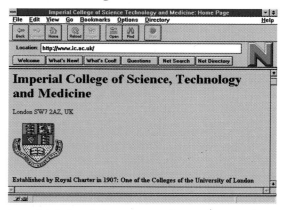

Imperial College's home page gives you access to a wide range of programs and shareware.

You can use the Internet to access computers that are dedicated to storing programs, pictures, sound, and video as well as text files. Some of these sites are open only to authorised users, but others allow anyone to dial in, browse, and download anything on offer. These are called anonymous FTP sites. One of the largest FTP sites in Britain is at Imperial College, London (ftp://src.doc.ic.ac.uk). To access the site simply type the address into the location box. Don't expect to find commercial programs, but there are extensive collections of shareware as well as many programs in the public domain which can all be obtained for the price of a local phone call.

## Newsgroups

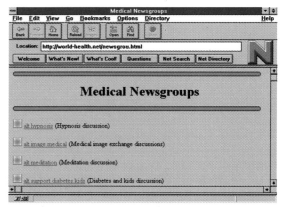

Johns Hopkins medical newsgroup list.

The Internet also lets you exchange news and views on a variety of subjects in forums called newsgroups. There are a growing number of groups dedicated to medical topics. Although they are of most interest to specialists, they are all open to the general public, and it is not uncommon to see a question posed by a patient with a problem. People using the system post messages or questions to a 24 hour global audience and can therefore expect several replies within a very short time. A list of current medical newsgroups is maintained at Johns Hopkins University (http://world-health.net/newsgrou.html). Some of these groups are very active, with hundreds of new messages being posted every day. If you intend to read and reply to these messages regularly it is a good idea to invest in a very fast modem.

---

### List of United Kingdom service providers

BBC Networking Club
| | |
|---|---|
| Demon | 0181 371 1234 |
| CompuServe | 0800 289378 |
| Nildram | 01442 891331 |
| UnipalmPipex UK | 01223 250120 |
| WinNET | 0181 863 1191 |

---

### Basic requirements to access the Internet

- Modern computer (PC or Macintosh) — £900
- Graphical User Interface—for example, Windows, OS/2, or Macintosh
- Modem 14 400 Baud (V32bis) or faster (V34) — £150
- Service provider
  - Start up cost — from £30
  - Monthly charges — from £10
  - Online charges — usually Nil
- Telephone line and call charges

The first figure is reproduced with permission of Kevin Hughes. All copyrights acknowledged.

# 11 ONLINE SEARCHING

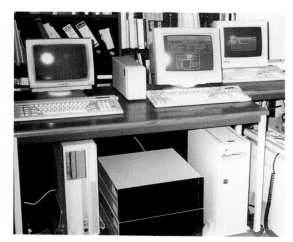

BMA's Medline system.

Searching for references is part of everyday life in medicine. If your computer is equipped with a modem and communications software you can now do online searches without needing to visit a library. Online searching refers to the use of information sources held on remote computer systems, perhaps the most popular of which is Medline.

The BMA library runs a Medline service for BMA members, which is available 24 hours a day through a modem and also through the Internet or Joint Academic Network (JANET). The Medline database runs on a modern PC with a very large hard disk in the library. The computer is connected to a number of telephone lines so up to 20 people can dial in and access the system simultaneously. BMA members can access the Medline database at no cost apart from normal telephone charges. You will, however, need to apply to the library for a password before using the system.

## Accessing the BMA library Medline system

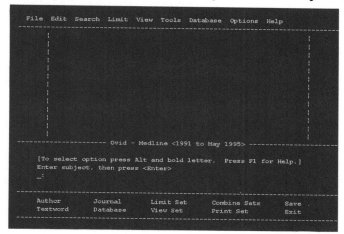

Initial search screen in Medline.

The following description is based on the OVID (3.0) DOS version of the system interface. It is best to use Norton pcAnywhere to access the BMA's Medline service as this gives best performance, but you can also use any standard communications program. The commands vary slightly depending on the program that you use but clear instructions are always given on the screen. When you log on to the database you need to type IBMOVID if you have Norton pcAnywhere or VTOVID if you have other communications software.

## Searching Medline

Results of a search for "heart attack".

To carry out a search on a particular subject, type the relevant term or phrase at the cursor prompt. The system will attempt to map your word(s) to relevant standard terms, known as medical subject headings (MeSH). Medline, which is produced by the United States National Library of Medicine, is indexed using over 17 500 such terms. They are designed to reduce problems that arise from, for example, use of synonyms and differences in British and American spelling. You will be asked to select the most appropriate term from those listed.

Once you have chosen an appropriate term the system will remind you of possible broader or narrower terms. The MeSH system has a tree structure in which broad subject terms branch into a series of progressively narrower subject terms.

## Online searching

```
-----------------Subheadings - Myocardial Infarction ----------------
+----------------------------------+  +------------------------------+
| |_| Include All Subheading _ 7493 |  | Subheadings will narrow a search |
| bl |_| Blood_____  349___ |  | to specific aspects of a topic. |
| ci |_| Chemically Induced___ 88__ |  |                                  |
| cl |_| Classification_____  3_ |  | Choosing 'Include All            |
| co |_| Complications_____ 700_ |  | Subheadings' will cause the      |
| di |_| Diagnosis_____ 717__ |  | system to retrieve all instances |
| dh |_| Diet Therapy_____ 15__ |  | of your subject heading no matter|
| dt |_| Drug Therapy_____ 1697_ |  | which subheading is applied, or  |
| ec |_| Economics_____  17__ |  | if no subheadings are applied.   |
| en |_| Enzymology_____  65__ |  |                                  |
| ep |_| Epidemiology_____ 233__ |  |                                  |
| eh |_| Ethnology_____  17__ |  |                                  |
| et |_| Etiology_____ 350__ |  |                                  |
| ge |_| Genetics_____ 63__ |  |                                  |
| hi |_| History_____  2__ |  |                                  |
| im |_| Immunology_____ 43  |  |                                  |
+----------------------------------+  +------------------------------+

   Use the spacebar to select one or more subheadings to apply to your term.

-------------------------------------------------------------------
        OK<Enter>   Previous   Cancel<Esc>   Help<F1>
-------------------------------------------------------------------
```

Subheadings allow you to tailor your search to your needs.

You can choose to search for a broad or very specific term. Alternatively, you can search for a broad term and then retrieve all related narrower terms by selecting the Explode option. All articles are indexed by using the most specific terms possible.

Next, you will be asked whether you wish the subject(s) chosen to be a main focus of the items retrieved. Choose Yes to increase the relevance of items retrieved on a well documented subject. After this you will be shown several subheadings associated with the term. Each term has about 80 subheadings in Medline indexing, which allows you to concentrate on particular aspects of the topic you have chosen.

# Main menu options

```
----------------------- Journal Name Index -------------------
-------------------------------------------------------------------
| jn | blood reviews                              |   106 |
| jn | blood vessels                              |    68 |
| jn | blutalkohol                                |   125 |
| jn | bmj                                        |  8479 |
| jn | boletin asociacion medica de puerto rico   |   185 |
| jn | boletin chileno de parasitologia           |    58 |
| jn | boletin de estudios medicos y biologicos   |    18 |
| jn | boletin de la oficina sanitaria panamericana|  139 |
| jn | boletin medico del hospital infantil de mexico| 331 |
| jn | bollettino chimico farmaceutico            |   161 |
| jn | bollettino dell istituto sieroterapico milanese| 22 |
| jn | bollettino societa italiana biologia sperimentale| 388 |
| jn | bone                                       |   375 |
| jn | bone & mineral                             |   389 |
| jn | bone marrow transplantation                |  1248 |
| jn | brain                                      |   465 |
-------------------------------------------------------------------

   Use the spacebar to select one or more terms to search.

-------------------------------------------------------------------
        OK<Enter>   Previous   Cancel<Esc>   Help<F1>
-------------------------------------------------------------------
```

The "Journal" option lets you look for articles published in a particular journal.

The Author and Journal options on the main menu let you select from a list of authors and journals. The Limit option will allow you to restrict a set of results in standard ways—for example, only English language or human subjects. Limits are applied cumulatively until you return to the main menu screen. The Combine option will allow you to bring together two or more sets of results. These may be combined using the Boolean operators and or or. Use and to combine sets in order to make your retrieved items more specific. Use or to merge sets to bring together similar concepts.

The Save option will allow you to save your current search strategy on the BMA host system or items retrieved to the hard or floppy disk of your own machine. The library's information pack contains detailed instructions on transferring search results to your computer. It is possible to download results for importing into a personal bibliographic software package such as Reference Manager or Pro-Cite.

```
---------------------------- Save Documents ------------------------
+-----------------------------------+  +-----------------------------+
| Save Name _:  hayfever            |  | Enter a 1-8 character file name to |
|                                   |  | identify this set of documents. |
| +Documents To Save--------------+ |  |                                 |
| | From _: 1      To _:    8     | |  | You can save All documents or   |
| |                               | |  | enter a range of document numbers. |
| | Preset Maximum:   1000        | |  | Both may be subject to a preset |
| |                               | |  | limit.                          |
| | Total in set:        8        | |  |                                 |
| +-------------------------------+ |  | Choose Floppy Drive to save your |
|                                   |  | documents to a portable diskette; |
|                                   |  | choose Hard Drive to save to the |
|                                   |  | hard drive (when available).     |
|                                   |  |                                 |
|                                   |  | Use the spacebar to select      |
|                                   |  | Include Strategy.  The strategy |
| [X]  Include Strategy             |  | will precede the documents.     |
+-----------------------------------+  +-----------------------------+

   Enter a 1-8 character Save Name and Tab to select items to modify.
   Tab to Options... to change the default fields, format or sort order.

-------------------------------------------------------------------
        OK<Enter>      Options...      Cancel<Esc>      Help<F1>
-------------------------------------------------------------------
```

The results of your search can be saved on your computer or a floppy disk.

The Textword option allows you to search for your own words or phrases in the titles and abstracts of records. This is useful, for example, if the subject for which you are searching is new and has not yet been given an indexing term, is a brand name, or is obscure. Retrieval for poorly documented subjects can sometimes be increased by combining a search for a text word with a search using indexing terms. Another useful technique is to check the MeSH terms for a relevant article already retrieved and to use these terms to trace further articles indexed in a similar way. With the old DOS interface there was a Find similar citations option which made this possible automatically while browsing. This is not yet available with the OVID interface. Use the Database option to change files (year bands) and repeat your search strategy in remaining files.

```
  File  View  Options  Tree  Help
-------------------- Tree Display - Eye Diseases -----------------
+--<+>Respiratory Tract Diseases                          | 1114
+--<+>Otorhinolaryngologic Diseases                      |  355
+--<+>Nervous System Diseases                            | 3165
+--<->Eye Diseases                                       | 1776
|  +--< >Asthenopia                                      |   56
|  +--<->Conjunctival Diseases                           |  227
|  |   +--< >Conjunctival Neoplasms                      |  158
|  |   +--<+>Conjunctivitis                              |  242
|  |   +--< >Pterygium                                   |  113
|  |   +--<X>Xerophthalmia                               |   88
|  +--<+>Corneal Diseases                                |  716
|  +--<+>Eye Abnormalities                               |  276
|  +--<+>Eye Diseases, Hereditary                        |   14
|  +--<+>Eye Hemorrhage                                  |   96
|  +--<+>Eye Infections                                  |  102
|  +--<+>Eye Injuries                                    |  548
-----------------------------------------------------------------
  Use the spacebar to select one or more terms to search.  Press plus <+>
  and minus <-> keys to expand and collapse terms.
-----------------------------------------------------------------
      Full Tree      Scope Note       Post Terms      Explode
      Contexts       Subheadings      New Term        Close
-----------------------------------------------------------------
```

The tree display shows the hierarchy of the MeSH headings.

```
  File  View  Options  Tree  Help
------------------- Permuted Index - lung ------------------
acute lung injury                                          |
     see RESPIRATORY DISTRESS SYNDROME, ADULT              |  123
BIRD FANCIER'S LUNG                                        |    3
budgerigar fancier's lung                                  |
     see BIRD FANCIER'S LUNG                               |    3
CARCINOMA, LEWIS LUNG                                      |    1
     see related MICE, INBRED C57BL                        |  980
CARCINOMA, NON-SMALL-CELL LUNG                             |  171
     see related LUNG NEOPLASMS                            | 1182
     see related CARCINOMA, SMALL CELL                     |  223
     see related ADENOCARCINOMA                            | 1044
     see related CARCINOMA, SQUAMOUS CELL                  |  816
     see related CARCINOMA, LARGE CELL                     |    5
     see related CARCINOMA, SMALL CELL                     |  223
carcinoma, small cell lung                                 |
     see CARCINOMA, SMALL CELL                             |  223
congenital cystic adenomatoid malformation of lung         |
-----------------------------------------------------------
  Use the spacebar to select one or more terms to search.
-----------------------------------------------------------
     Post Terms   Explode   Scope Note   Tree   New Term   Close
-----------------------------------------------------------
```

With the permuted index you can find all the MeSH headings containing a particular word.

Choosing Tree from the Tools menu, in the top section of the initial search screen will allow you to check the tree position of a particular MeSH term. Choosing Permuted Index will allow you to check, alphabetically, on the MeSH terms which contain a particular word. This is especially useful as MeSH terms can be single words or phrases and, when phrases, may not follow conventional word order (for example, "Neoplasms, Multiple Primary"). In either case the Scope Note option will offer guidance on the use of the MeSH terms selected.

*Searching without menus*

It is possible to put in search commands directly at the cursor prompt on the main menu screen. To search for a term in a particular field throughout the database enter the chosen term plus the two letter label for the field to be searched—for example, asthma.ti to search for the word "asthma" in the title. To search for a particular word stem in titles throughout the database use $—for example, child$.ti would find children as well as child. However, if you cut back the search stem too far many irrelevant items could be retrieved.

The back search command is available through the old DOS interface but not the OVID system. This enables you to repeat a search carried out in the most recent file of the database throughout the remaining files, as one operation, and will provide a combined result. Having carried out your search, type ..bs at the cursor prompt.

# Bath Information and Data Service (BIDS)

## Main databases available from BIDS

- Citation Indexes (ISI)—Three indexes (Science Citation Index (SCI), Social Science Citation Index (SSCI), and Arts and Humanities Citation Index (A&HCI)) covering 7500 journals dating back to 1981. References of the indexed articles can be searched as well. Articles, editorials, letters, and reviews are all indexed
- Index to Scientific and Technical Proceedings (ISTP)—Contains information on published proceedings for about 4200 conferences a year including details of individual papers
- Embase—Covers 3500 biomedical journals from 110 countries with good coverage of drugs and toxicology. Two thirds of the articles have abstracts and the abstract text is searchable
- Inside Information—From the British Library Document Supply Centre. It covers details of every major article in 10 000 of their most requested titles. One million articles are added each year
- Ei Compendex*Plus—An engineering database including medical engineering. It covers 2600 international journals. Entries are taken from journal articles, technical reports, conference papers, and proceedings
- Ei Page One—Gives contents pages of 5400 journals
- IBSS Online—International Bibliography of the Social Sciences supplied by the British Library of Political and Economic Science at the London School of Economics. Covers 2600 international social science journals and 6000 books
- UnCover—Database of current articles from over 15 000 journals with a brief description on each article. It enables contents pages of journals to be created and allows articles to be sent directly to your fax machine

Although Medline is one of the most popular databases used by healthcare professionals, several other medically oriented databases are available which allow you to widen the scope of your search. Some of these other databases are connected to a common access point based in Bath—the Bath Information and Data Service (BIDS).

BIDS is designed to be used by non-expert searchers, but you may find it useful to ask for a demonstration before you use it for the first time. BIDS supplies excellent leaflets about its databases which guide you through the service, and once logged on you can also obtain context sensitive help at any time by simply typing Help. A detailed self help guide is available which contains many worked practical examples. Information about BIDS is also available on the Internet (http://www.bids.ac.uk).

# Online searching

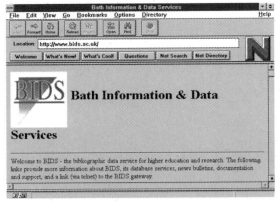

BIDS Internet home page.

```
         /
  BBBB   IIIII  DDDD    SSS
  B   B    I    D   D   S               Bath Information
  BBBB     I    D   D   SSS
  B   B    I    D   D       S           and Data Services
  B   B    I    D   D   S   S
  BBBB   IIIII  DDDD    SSS
 /
/  /
/    Please type the option number for the service you require:

Option   Service                Option   Service
------   -------                ------   -------
  1      BIDS EMBASE              5       BIDS Ecoflora
  2      BIDS ISI                 6       Blackwell's UnCover
  3      BIDS BL Inside Information 7     BIDS IBSS
  4      BIDS Compendex/Page One

  n      News                   q or x   Quit from this gateway
  h or ? Help
```

Starting to search the Embase database.

```
BIDS EMBASE Service

*** UNAUTHORISED USE IS PROHIBITED ***

Username: IABC1234
Password:
_____

                    -- BIDS EMBASE --

  1  Search EMBASE database
  2  Show news
  3  Show local information
  4  Show introduction to EMBASE
  5  Show legal agreement
```

Search menu in Embase.

```
Current (->) article number 1 of 773 is unmarked
->TI: The economics of depression in primary care. Department of Health
      initiatives
  AU: Lloyd_K, Jenkins_R
  JN: British Journal of Psychiatry, 1995, Vol.166, No.APR. S27, pp.60-62

  TI: CD8+ and CD45RA+ human peripheral blood lymphocytes are potent
      sources of macrophage inflammatory protein 1alpha interleukin-8 and
      RANTES
  AU: Conlon_K, Lloyd_A, Chattopadhyay_U, Lukacs_N, Kunkel_S, Schall_T,
      Taub_D, Morimoto_C, Osborne_J, Oppenheim_J, Young_H, Kelvin_D,
      Ortaldo_J
  JN: European Journal of Immunology, 1995, Vol.25, No.3, pp.751-756

  TI: Psychiatric and social outcome of liver transplantation
  AU: Collis_I, Burroughs_A, Rolles_K, Lloyd_G
  JN: British Journal of Psychiatry, 1995, Vol.166, No.APR., pp.521-524

-----------------------------------------------------------------------
UP/DOWN arrow keys to scroll, RETURN for next page,
SPACE to mark/unmark current article, Q to quit display
-----------------------------------------------------------------------
or Search(S) Display(D) Output(P) Options(O) Issues(I) Thesaurus(T) Order(B)
or type HELP or EXIT
```

Display of search results restricted to title, author, and journal.

## How to connect to BIDS

Most academic libraries and computer centres connected to the Internet or to JANET should be able to provide access to BIDS. To use the system you need to ask the library to give you a username and password. BIDS also provides access to the Blackwell UnCover service, which is free to any member of staff or student of an institution which has subscribed to BIDS. It requires no username or password. Each of the other databases in the BIDS system has to be subscribed to separately. However, once your institution has taken out a subscription it is free to individual users.

## Searching for information

After connecting to BIDS you will be presented with a menu from which you have to choose a database to search. The system allows you to search only one database at a time. Once the database has been selected you will be asked to enter your username and password. You should then select the search the database option from the initial menu, which brings up the search menu.

The next step is to choose a field to search in—for example, title, author, or key words. The search term can be a single word, a phrase, or an expression linked with the logical operators and, or, and not. The screen will tell you how many references have been retrieved. If there is more than one the Display and Output options appear at the bottom of the search menu screen. To view your results press D followed by the return key, which brings up the display menu. You can choose how much detail is displayed, ranging from titles only to full records including authors' addresses, abstract, text, etc.

Instead of noting down details from the screen you can send the results to your email box by choosing the Output option. Your local computing service should be able to give you an email number, which you will have to enter every time you want search results sent to you.

BIDS can provide simultaneous access to only a limited number of users, and it is a popular service. It is therefore important to plan your search before you start to ensure that you are logged on for the minimum possible time. If your search runs into problems it is probably best to leave the system by typing Exit. You can then rethink your search strategy and take advice from your librarian or BIDS before trying again.

## Refining the search strategy

Each search is recorded in a search history table. Search strategies can then be reused and combined to search multiple fields—for example, title, abstract, author, or institution. Using several fields narrows the search and reduces the number of inappropriate references retrieved. It is also easy to reuse search strategies saved during a previous session. If necessary these can be modified or combined before running them again.

You can also search using the Embase thesaurus facility. Entering T (for Thesaurus) brings up a dialogue box where you can either enter an exact thesaurus term or perform a "fuzzy match" search against all the registered thesaurus terms. Once you have settled on a term you can carry out simple searches, do explosion searches (searching all the branches of the thesaurus tree), include or exclude looking for the term in the minor keywords field; you can also qualify your search with drug or disease subheadings.

There are several ways to modify the scope of searches. Firstly, you can change the range of years from the default (three plus the current year) to any range back to the beginning of the data (1980). Secondly, you can limit the search to any material added since any arbitrary date in the last six months or to material added since a saved search question was last run. Searches can also be restricted to articles published in selected languages, and you can select (or exclude) particular document types such as articles, letters, or reviews.

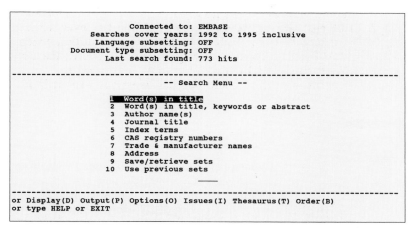

```
                   Connected to: EMBASE
        Searches cover years: 1992 to 1995 inclusive
           Language subsetting: OFF
      Document type subsetting: OFF
           Last search found: 773 hits

-----------------------------------------------------------------------
                        -- Search Menu --

           1  Word(s) in title
           2  Word(s) in title, keywords or abstract
           3  Author name(s)
           4  Journal title
           5  Index terms
           6  CAS registry numbers
           7  Trade & manufacturer names
           8  Address
           9  Save/retrieve sets
          10  Use previous sets

-----------------------------------------------------------------------
or Display(D) Output(P) Options(O) Issues(I) Thesaurus(T) Order(B)
or type HELP or EXIT
```

Searches can be refined to increase relevance of references retrieved.

*Other facilities*

The BIDS system allows you to mark a selection of articles of interest from all those retrieved for subsequent display or output. Copies of the original article can also be ordered from a supplier such as the British Library Document Supply Centre. A replica of the contents page of a particular journal issue can be obtained by using the Issues menu.

When you have completed your search you should leave the system by typing exit and pressing the return key. Any results that you emailed will then need to be retrieved from your email box. You can then print these in the library or copy them on to a floppy disk for transfer into your own computer. The library or computing service will advise you on how to do this.

**Useful contacts**

BMA Library Free Medline
    Service                    0171 383 6224
Bath Information and Data
    Services (BIDS) Helpdesk 01225 826074
BIDS Internet homepage    http://www.bids.ac.uk

# 12  BIBLIOGRAPHIC SOFTWARE

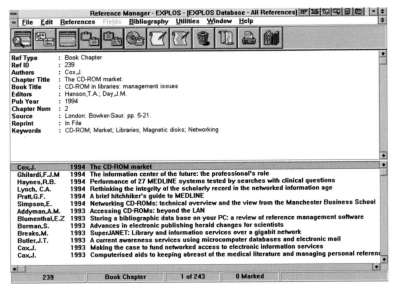

Bibliographic software helps organise your references.

Biomedical literature has expanded rapidly in recent years. Over 300 000 new articles are added to the Medline database each year, and this is just one of many computerised databases. Doctors doing literature searches with these databases commonly find more than 100 references on a specific subject. The challenge is to manage this flow of information efficiently so that key references can easily be stored on your personal computer and located some months later when you need to use them. Several bibliographic reference databases have been developed to meet this challenge. They allow large numbers of references to be stored, indexed, and retrieved easily.

## Creating a reference database

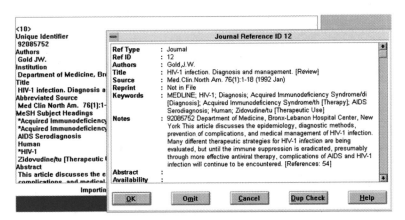

References from Medline are automatically converted into the format used by the bibliographic software.

References are managed in bibliographic software packages by storing them in groups of related subjects. The software automatically takes care of the structuring necessary to accommodate a range of different reference types—for example, journal articles, book chapters, abstracts.

### Importing data or references

Although you can type references into the database using the menus and prompts provided, it is far easier to import them electronically from other sources. Most libraries offer facilities which allow you to copy references from CD ROMs, or you could dial into a remote database such as Medline in the BMA Library. When importing data electronically the bibliographic software automatically converts references from the native format into that required by the program. This eliminates the tedium of typing and reduces the risk of transcription errors.

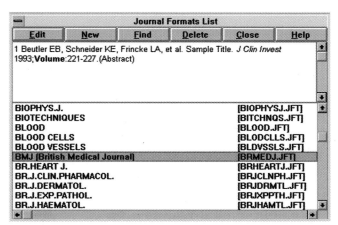

Reference Manager will show you the style required by the main medical journals.

Fast and flexible retrieval of specific references is essential, especially as the database grows. The software lets you search for references by the name of an author, a word in the title of an article, or the name of a journal. Different combinations of terms can be searched by linking them through the "and", "or", and "not" operators. Thus a search for "kidney and transplantation" will find only those references in which both terms occur.

### Managing reprints

Bibliographic software can also help you keep track of any reprints that you might have obtained. Some packages include a field in which it is possible to indicate if a reprint is held for a given reference and, if so, where the reprint is filed.

# Generation of a bibliography

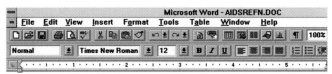

**Progress in AIDS Diagnosis**

A recent review of the diagnosis and management of HIV infection[1] reported that....

Bibliography

1 Gold JW. HIV-1 infection. Diagnosis and management. *Med Clin North Am* 1992;**76**:1-18.

References can be converted to the required style simply by clicking a button.

For anyone who publishes papers regularly the most valued feature of bibliographic software is the facility to create a list of references which can be appended to a manuscript. The publishers of medical journals and books all have their own specifications about the way in which references should be formatted—for example, Vancouver or Harvard styles. Most of the software packages will automatically produce the reference list in several different styles to meet the requirements of the major journals. Furthermore, the software will also place appropriate reference numbers in the text of your manuscript. These features take much of the drudgery out of preparing a paper.

---

### Features of bibliographic software

Allows creation of groups of related articles— for example, one for AIDS and one for tuberculosis

Automatic incorporation of data or references from other sources such as Medline

Easy retrieval of data or references

Management of reprints

Generates lists of references in all standard formats for inclusion in paper

---

### Bibliographic software

| | |
|---|---|
| Reference Manager—Costly but aimed specifically at medical market | 01895 813544 |
| EndNote—Strong on generating bibliographies, but aimed at humanities rather than medicine | 01865 784800 |
| Pro-Cite—Very powerful but expensive | 01865 326612 |
| Papyrus—Good value for money, but onus is on user to develop routines for importing data | 01960 351532 |

# 13 CD ROMS, MULTIMEDIA, AND OPTICAL STORAGE SYSTEMS

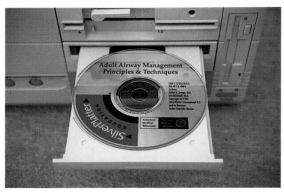

CD ROM drive.

CD ROMs (compact disc read only memory) have emerged as one of the most useful technologies of the 1990s. They look identical to the familiar audio compact disc, but store large amounts of computer data rather than music. Fortunately, they are as easy to use as their audio counterparts. Prices start at just a few pounds, although subscriptions to some of the medical databases can be expensive (about £1000 a year).

To access these titles you need a CD ROM drive in your computer. If necessary, these drives are easy to install, but they are increasingly found as a standard fitting on many new computers.

## Text only disks

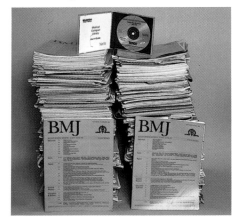

Macmillan's Medical Compact Library.

Each CD ROM has a capacity of over 600 megabytes—equivalent to more than 400 floppy disks—and can store up to 300 000 pages of text. They are therefore ideal for storing articles published in medical journals. The disc shown opposite contains every article published in the *BMJ* over the past seven years (over 17 000). Another disc in the same series contains every article published over the past year in the *Lancet*, *BMJ*, *Annals of Internal Medicine*, *New England Journal of Medicine*, and *JAMA*. SilverPlatter produces several text based CD ROMs covering a wide range of medical topics. For example, the AIDSLINE disc contains over 99 000 records from 1980 to the present taken from over 3000 journals, plus government reports, letters, technical reports, abstracts and papers from meetings, monographs, special publications, and theses. Any of these discs can easily be searched for a specific word or phrase. Any relevant articles that you find can then be printed out or viewed on the screen.

## Multimedia

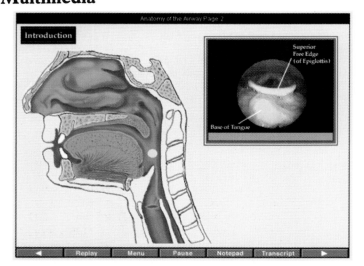

SilverPlatter's CD ROM *Adult Airway Management*. Clicking on pictures will sometimes run a short video.

More complex CD ROM titles containing a rich mixture of text, colour photographs, video clips, animations, and stereo sound are now being released. These are known as multimedia CD ROMs. Using a multimedia disc is similar to watching a documentary on television except that you can choose exactly what you want to see and hear next. Many new medical multimedia titles are published each month. They have added a completely new dimension to undergraduate and postgraduate teaching. Many of these discs end with a multiple choice examination and print off a "report". In some countries this can be submitted as evidence of having undertaken continuing medical education.

# Photo CD

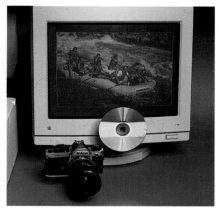

Photo CDs let you store pictures for later use in slides and printed reports.

Photo CD is a system developed by Kodak which allows you to transfer up to 100 colour photographs taken on a standard 35 mm camera on to a special CD ROM. You need to purchase a blank disc from a photographic dealer and send it to the processors along with the film. After development the photographs are scanned electronically and stored on the disc, which is then returned to you along with the slides or prints. If there is room left on the disc, further photographs can be added at a later date. The photo CD can be used in any PC or Macintosh equipped with a multisession CD ROM drive and suitable software. The stored images can easily be incorporated into your documents by using a desktop publishing program or word processor and into slides with a presentation graphics program. You can also purchase prerecorded Photo CDs containing several royalty free medical images.

# Installing a CD ROM drive

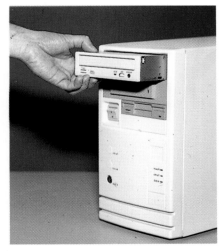

Installing a CD ROM drive.

## Hardware

Most CD ROM drives are fitted internally into a $5\frac{1}{4}''$ drive bay at the front of the computer, although external drives are also available for notebooks or computers without a free drive bay. The CD ROM drive is connected to the computer via an interface card. Until recently, most plugged into a sound card but newer drives connect to a standard IDE socket alongside the hard disk. If you wish to use multimedia a stereo sound card and either headphones or hi-fi loudspeakers are essential. Installing a drive and sound card is very simple and does not require any special knowledge or tools. Despite this, many people prefer to have the drive fitted by the computer dealer.

## Software

You will also need to install software which allows the computer and CD ROM drive to communicate. Most drives are supplied with a floppy disk which contains all the necessary programs. Follow the manufacturer's instructions to copy the programs from the floppy on to your hard disk. The speed and usability of CD ROM drives, especially older models, is greatly enhanced by disk caching software. A suitable program called Smartdrive is supplied free with MSDOS, although only the later versions recognise CD ROM drives.

# Using a CD ROM drive

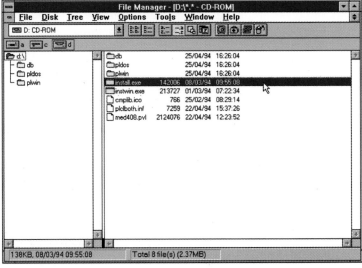

Directory listing of a CD ROM.

Once the drive is installed a CD ROM is used in exactly the same way as a floppy or hard disk. The CD ROM drive is usually automatically assigned a drive letter during installation (normally the next letter after the hard disk). For example, if the hard disk is drive C the CD ROM will be assigned drive D. To change to the CD ROM, type D: and press the enter key. Programs can often be run directly from the CD ROM, but it is more usual to install programs on to your system. During installation key program files are copied on to your hard disk, where they run more quickly, but all large files (pictures, sounds, movies) are normally left on the CD ROM. Despite the fact that CD ROMs store large amounts of data, some databases require several discs. In these cases the program will prompt you to change discs when necessary.

## Playing audio compact discs

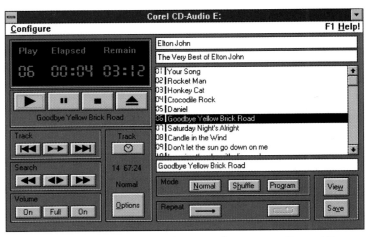

Corel CD Audio gives you control over audio compact discs while you work on something else.

Most CD ROM drives allow you to play standard audio compact discs while working on something else (for example, a word processor). You listen to the music through headphones or loudspeakers plugged into the computer. A simple program is needed to control the compact disc. This is almost always included on the floppy disk supplied in the CD ROM package, although you might need to copy it to the hard disk manually.

Windows 3.11 includes a simple program (Media Player), although there are others (for example, Corel CD Audio) which offer much more control and which automatically display not only the title but also the tracks of the compact disc. Windows 95 will automatically play music compact discs as soon as they are inserted.

## Recordable disks

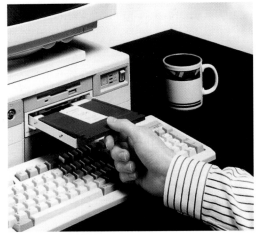

Panasonic PD drive.

Standard CD ROM drives are "read only," which means that it is not possible to record your own data on to the disk. Recordable drives and discs (CD-R) are available but are mainly used by organisations wishing to distribute large amounts of information in the CD ROM format to a relatively small number of people. They remain expensive and the disks are not as robust as other rewritable optical disks.

A hybrid system—the Panasonic PD drive—lets you read ordinary CD ROMs and record data on to special blank rewritable disks with a capacity of 650 megabytes. Unfortunately, these special disks can be played back only in another PD drive and cannot be used in a standard CD ROM drive. The PD drive will probably be most useful in top of the range computers, particularly those designed as graphics workstations, where storage requirements are large and cheap bulk storage important.

## Other optical storage systems

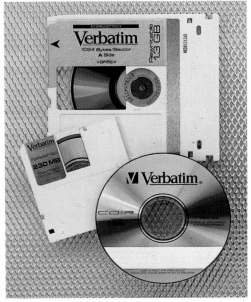

Rewritable optical disks.

### Rewritable optical disk drives

These drives and disks are manufactured in two formats: $3\frac{1}{2}''$ and $5\frac{1}{4}''$. The disks have maximum capacities of 230 megabytes and 1·3 gigabytes respectively, although this is likely to increase in the future. All modern drives are backwardly compatible and can read disks recorded in older drives. Rewritable drives use one of two different technologies to write to the disks (magneto-optical and phase change).

Optical systems are slower than modern magnetic hard disks but have several advantages over magnetic systems. Most importantly, they have a very large storage capacity and the disks are robust and immune to damage from stray magnetic fields. Many manufacturers of optical systems guarantee the integrity of stored data for 30 years. Although the drives are expensive, the disks are cheap, which makes them ideal if you need to store large amounts of data—for example, for document image processing (DIP) and in a graphics workstation. You can use an unlimited number of disks in a drive and, as they are removable, they can be locked up in a safe overnight for added security against fire or theft. For this reason, they are sometimes used as an alternative to tape based backup systems

## Applications benefiting from optical storage

- Data backup
- Software distribution
- Multimedia applications
- Document image processing
- Medical and general information databases
- Medical image storage—for example, photographs, radiographs

### WORM drives

WORM drives (write once read many times) are a variant of the rewritable drives described above. The difference is that data cannot be changed once written to the disk. This kind of system has obvious advantages in situations where an audit trail is essential. They are used in several financial institutions but are not commonly found in medical computers, although they have been used in some dental practice systems.

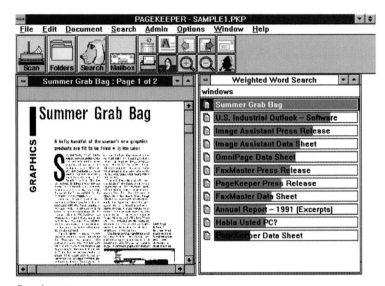

Pagekeeper.

### Document image processing (DIP)

Many large organisations have eliminated paper records by using document image processing. All incoming mail is scanned electronically. The text is read by optical character recognition (OCR) software then automatically indexed and stored along with an electronic image of the original document. Anyone permitted access to the system can then rapidly search through every document in the system for a particular word or phrase. Charts and pictures can also be stored and viewed. Several people can access the same document simultaneously. If necessary, the image of the original documents can be laser printed on to paper. The quality is similar to that of a good photocopy. Although there are many advantages in using such a system (not least the elimination of bulky paper records), they raise some unresolved medicolegal issues. The storage requirements for this type of system are so large that optical disks are the only realistic option.

### Useful telephone numbers

| | | |
|---|---|---|
| SilverPlatter | Free directory of electronic resources on CD ROM | 0800 262096 |
| Macmillan | Medical compact library (*BMJ* on CD ROM etc) | 001 617 661 2955 |
| SSVC | SilverPlatter multimedia medical training CD ROM | 0831 596759 |
| Kodak | Information on Photo CD system | 01442 61122 |
| Caere Corp | PageKeeper UK Information Centre | 0171 222 3200 |
| Focus 77 | Comprehensive catalogue of medical CD ROMs | 0500 947177 |
| | The Medical Directory CD ROM | 0171 896 2424 |

# 14  USING COMPUTERS IN CLINICAL AUDIT

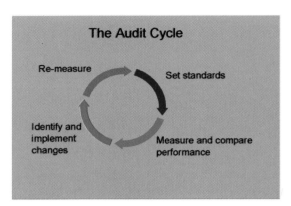

**The Audit Cycle**

Set standards → Measure and compare performance → Identify and implement changes → Re-measure

---

**Clinical audit**

The systematic critical analysis of the quality of care, including the procedures used for diagnosis and treatment, the use of resources, and the resulting outcome and quality of life for the patient.

---

Clinical audit is generally described as a cycle composed of several stages, the traditional audit cycle. Put simply, it is a way of improving current performance by deciding on the ideal (setting standards), looking at the real situation (measuring current performance), and finding ways of moving from the real to the ideal (implementing change). The cycle is closed by reassessing performance after an interval to assess the effectiveness of the change.

All clinicians should be measuring their performance against a locally defined standard. In addition, as awareness of the usefulness of audit increases other issues about guidelines are being raised. There is a growing move towards evidence based medicine and a feeling that best practice can be agreed nationally (or internationally) and local standards developed from guidelines. It is therefore becoming increasingly important to collect clinical information in a way that allows it to be pooled for both local and national analysis. Computers are ideally suited to this role.

## Computers and audit

---

**Advantages and disadvantages of using a computer for audit**

| Advantages | Disadvantages |
| --- | --- |
| Handle large amount of data | Difficult to use |
| Rapid retrieval of data | Require extensive training |
| Rapid analysis of data | Regarded as "black holes" where data disappear |
| Automated quality control as data are entered | Data extracted only as good as that put in (garbage in, garbage out) |
| Automatic production of reports | Data must be accurate, reliable, valid, complete, and timely |
| Legible records | Planning required before implementing |
| Records can be accessed by more than one person at a time | |
| Data for epidemiology readily available | |

---

For many people audit has become synonymous with computers. This idea was reinforced when a large proportion of the money ringfenced for audit was spent on computer systems, with varying degrees of success.

Audit is about asking questions concerning clinical practice and necessitates analysis of clinical data. For a few cases, or small data sets, this can be achieved with paper based systems, and many successful audits have not used computers at all. However, if you have a large data set or large numbers of cases paper based systems become difficult to use. Computers are excellent tools for storing and handling large amounts of data, and they can sort through, retrieve, and analyse data in a fraction of the time it takes to do it on paper.

## Computerised audit systems

---

**Examples of routine computerised systems**

General practice systems
Nursing systems
Case mix systems
Departmental systems
Clinical information systems (CIS)
Patient administration systems (PAS)
Resource management systems (RM)
Hospital information support systems (HISS)

---

Every audit project will be different, depending on the setting, the data to be collected, the people collecting the data, the timescale, the analysis required, and the involvement of information technologists. However, computer systems used in audit projects can be loosely categorised into three classes—routine systems, specialised systems, and ad hoc locally produced systems.

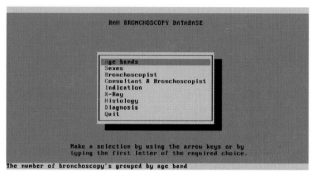

```
 A Add an Audit           P Perform an Audit
 R Audit Results          D Delete an Audit
 E Edit Audit             V View Parameters
 S Slide Dates            N Run Audit Nightly
 B Build/Edit audit reports

   Title
A Disease Incidence Audit from 1/4/90 to 1/4/91
  Dates relate to 1.4.91     Performed on 23.6.94
B Consultations from April 90 to April 91
  Dates relate to 1.4.91     Performed on 13.1.95
C Referral Audit for 1/4/91
  Dates relate to 1.4.91     Performed on 13.1.95
D 5 Year Old Immunisation Audit on 1/4/91
  Dates relate to 1.4.91     Performed on 13.1.95
E 2 Year Old Immunisation Audit for 1/4/91
  Dates relate to 1.4.91     Performed on 13.1.95
F Cervical Smear Audit on 1/4/91
  Dates relate to 1.4.91     Performed on 13.1.95
Select menu option  :            <Pg Up><PgDn>
```

General practice systems offer sophisticated audit facilities.

```
          RAH BRONCHOSCOPY DATABASE

        ┌─────────────────────────────┐
        │ Age bands                   │
        │ Sexes                       │
        │ Bronchoscopist              │
        │ Consultant & Bronchoscopist │
        │ Indication                  │
        │ X-Ray                       │
        │ Histology                   │
        │ Diagnosis                   │
        │ Quit                        │
        └─────────────────────────────┘

      Make a selection by using the arrow keys or by
        typing the first letter of the required choice.

The number of bronchoscopy's grouped by age band
```

A bronchoscopy database.

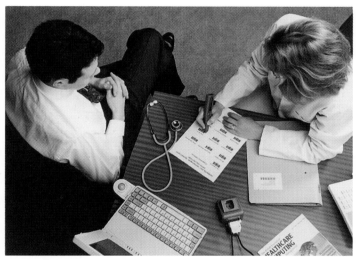

Bar code reader.

```
   ...  Referral Audit Database  ...
                                       04/04

Patient Number:        1254

Patient Name:          JOHN SMITH

Date of Referral:      12/03/95

Date Seen:             24/08/95

Referral Type:         S      (Options can be U,H,S)

Name of Referrer:      DR GREEN

Specialty:             PHYSIOTHERAPY

Referred to Named Individual:  Y



Write data to disk (Y/N)?
<Ctrl-N>-New <Ctrl-F>-Find F5-Print F6-Delete F9-Choices F10-Done  Rec=   1
```

A locally produced database.

## Routine systems

Many different and incompatible computer systems have been developed for use in the NHS. These often require a sophisticated and expensive information technology infrastructure and were usually designed for administration rather than audit. They have been introduced with varying degrees of involvement of clinical staff, with the result that many clinicians do not use them. These systems can, however, be a rich source of data for audit, although it may first be necessary to link up with information stored in separate administrative or departmental databases. This potential has not been exploited in the past, although information technologists running these systems are often able to help extract useful information.

## Specialised audit systems

These commercial systems are designed specially for audit and run on individual computers or small departmental networks. Some are able to extract information such as name, address, date of birth, general practitioner, and basic clinical data from existing routine systems. This saves time and reduces the risk of error in transcription. However, the systems can be inflexible and difficult or expensive to change, especially if outside help is required to produce reports for new audits.

The software is often accompanied by hardware devices such as bar code and optical mark readers. These can be used to collect large amounts of data rapidly and accurately, and they save much time. Bar codes, similar to those used in supermarkets, are assigned to each patient, event, or procedure, and a bar code reader is used to enter data into the system without the need for any typing. Optical mark readers are used in conjunction with specially devised forms, which are marked by the person seeing the patient. Information on the forms is then automatically scanned into the system.

## Locally produced systems

With a little technical knowledge you can set up databases or spreadsheets for use in small scale local audit projects. Such systems have the advantage of being very flexible and can be modified as the needs of the audit change. It can, however, be very time consuming to design and create such a system and it will always lack the advantage of feedback from a wide user base. The lack of a sophisticated interface sometimes makes them difficult for members of staff to use. Furthermore, it is difficult to connect them directly to other routine systems, and transferring data manually can lead to inaccuracies.

# Coding systems

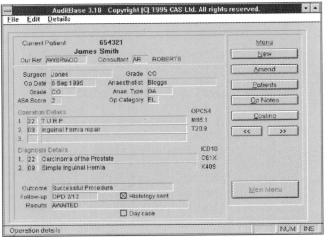

Hospital based audit system using OPCS and ICD codes.

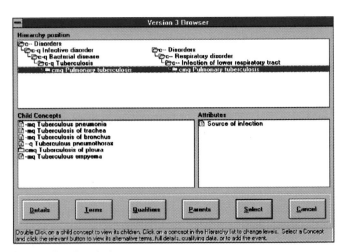

Mapping codes between Read and ICD 10.

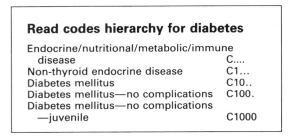

Clinicians sometimes use the same word or phrase (such as chest infection or dyspepsia) to describe a variety of conditions or several different terms for the same condition (for example, heart attack and myocardial infarction). The term used largely depends on personal preference. If these ambiguous terms are used in computer systems, confusion can arise when data are retrieved for audit or research. For this reason several coding systems have been developed to remove the ambiguity. Systems that use a coding system have the added advantage that the data they contain can be pooled for multicentre, national, or international audit and research.

*Read codes*

The most commonly used clinical coding systems are the International Classification of Diseases (ICD), which is used by many hospitals to claim payment from purchasing authorities, and Office of Population Censuses and Surveys (OPCS), which is used for statistical returns to the government and by the insurance industry. Neither of these systems offers enough codes to enable the creation of comprehensive clinical records. Read codes were therefore developed to enable electronic patient records to hold a huge range of clinical concepts in a concise, compact and unambiguous form. Although initially developed for use in general practice, they have been adopted by the Department of Health for use in the whole of the NHS.

*Read code hierarchy*

The Read code system is organised using a hierarchy of clinical terms which offers great advantages in clinical audit or research. For example, searches for the broad terms "respiratory disorder" or "infective disorder" will both find a patient with pulmonary tuberculosis. The core terms are updated quarterly to keep pace with changing clinical practice and drug terms are updated monthly. A recent update has added qualifying terms which can be recorded alongside the core term to add extra detail, such as left or right side.

You do not need to learn or use Read codes as computer systems using them are designed to allow the relevant term to be entered as text. The software will automatically look up the term in a thesaurus, identify the relevant core term, and record the appropriate code along with any qualifiers. You never see the code itself.

Typical Read code browser.

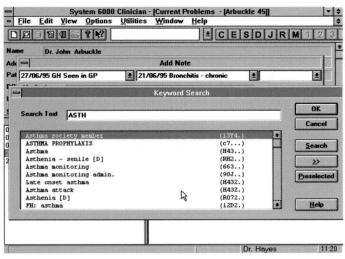

Adding a new problem to a general practice computer system.

*The future*

Since about 90% of general practices in Britain are already computerised and the Department of Health has insisted that all general practice computer systems use Read codes, detailed information about consultations, diseases, treatments, and outcomes relating to 50 million patients is already potentially available in a comparable electronic format. When the remaining practices are computerised, Read codes have been adopted by hospital based systems, and the NHS-wide network has been completed, there will be an unparalleled opportunity to undertake comprehensive, national audits and epidemiological research.

## Some clinical audit systems

| Company | System | Description | Phone No |
|---|---|---|---|
| AAH Meditel | System 5 | General practice routine system with audit capabilities | 01527 579414 |
| Chameleon Information Management Services | InfoMan | | 0181 954 5202 |
| Clinical Audit Systems Ltd | AuditBase | Windows based hospital audit system developed by clinicians | 01989 768717 |
| Clinical Computing UK | Proton, Abies CIS | Multispecialty clinical information systems with audit capabilities | 0181 742 7400 |
| Compucorp | Maisy | Windows-based multispecialty, administration and audit | 0181 907 0198 |
| Egton Medical Information Systems | EMIS | General practice routine system with audit capabilities | 0113 258 2454 |
| First Data Health Systems (UK) | First decision | Hospital-wide system with inbuilt audit capabilities | 01628 470800 |
| Healthcare Computer Systems | Auditman | Departmental and hospital-wide systems with audit modules available | 01733 558919 |
| ICS Medical | Clinics | Clinical information system with audit capabilities | 0161 480 7768 |
| Medical Systems | Micromed | Clinical information and audit system | 01494 866031 |
| Metasa | Metabase | Clinical data management and audit system | 01932 779977 |
| Siemens Nixdorf Information Systems | CaMIS clinical support system | Used in conjunction with case mix system and departmental systems for audit | 01344 862222 |
| VAMP Health | VAMP | General practice routine system with audit capabilities | 0171 498 1330 |

# 15 CLINICAL COMPUTER SYSTEMS IN GENERAL PRACTICE

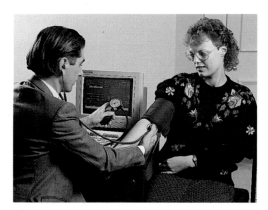

General practice consultation.

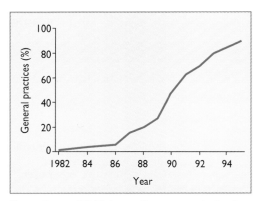

Percentage of British practices computerised.

General practitioners have been at the forefront of medical computing in Britain for the past 20 years. The first systems were developed by enthusiasts and were designed to collect epidemiological data rather than manage the practice, but in 1972 the Department of Health sponsored the development of a system that recorded consultations for the first time. The project was limited to a small group of practices in Exeter but subsequently developed into a full practice management system that is still available today. In 1982 another government sponsored scheme (Micros for GPs) put computers into 150 practices across the country, but it was not until 1987, when two companies (VAMP and Meditel) began offering sophisticated computer systems to general practitioners free of charge, that practice computing really took off.

In return for their free computers general practitioners were required to record every consultation and prescription issued. Both companies planned to collect this information anonymously and then sell it to pharmaceutical companies to recover their investment. From the general practitioners' perspective, the schemes were a huge success, stimulating many practices to computerise for the first time.

The sweeping changes to remuneration introduced in the 1990 general practice contract made computers almost essential for all but the smallest practices. By 1993 there were about 50 commercial systems to choose from and about 8500 practices were fully computerised. The free schemes have now ended, but the government continues to encourage computerisation through a complex system of reimbursement.

## Modern general practice systems

### Features of modern general practice systems

**Basic features:**

**Age-sex register**
**Comprehensive clinical records**
**Acute and repeat prescribing**
**Call and recall systems**
**Complex reporting modules for**
   **Practice management**
   **Clinical audit**
**Word processing linked to database**
**Email between users**
**Electronic links to family health services**
   **authorities and hospital pathology**
   **laboratories**

**Optional extras:**

Appointment systems
Fundholding software
Various "expert systems"
Portable computers for home visits

The competing general practice systems vary greatly but they do share several common features. All have evolved into advanced practice management tools that allow practices to run more efficiently. Furthermore, the systems now contain extraordinary amounts of information on patients and disease, with more being added every day. This unique source of epidemiological information has yet to be tapped, but the Department of Health has been steadily influencing the development of the systems so that it will eventually be possible to pool clinical data for national audit and research. General practice systems are likely to make an important contribution towards the development of evidence based medicine.

Most current general practice systems are built around a central computer (containing the processor, memory, and hard disk) connected to a series of terminals (screen and keyboard) in the reception area, offices, and all consulting rooms. These "dumb" terminals have no built in processor but use the power of the central computer. As a result, they do not need a noisy cooling fan—a great advantage during consultations. However, at busy times (for example, during morning surgery) when several people use the computer simultaneously response times can slow dramatically.

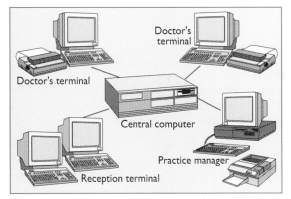

Typical general practice computing system.

Most general practitioners' terminals are attached directly to a prescription printer in the consulting room, while office terminals use plain paper printers (such as a laser printer) for letters and reports. The reception area usually has a printer dedicated to repeat prescriptions. Practice managers often use a DOS or Windows workstation to run business applications such as spreadsheets or payroll programs. Practices with a branch surgery may lease a dedicated telephone line to carry computer signals to and from the main surgery. Among other advantages, this allows any patient's record to be accessed from either surgery, but such sophisticated links are expensive to maintain.

## Registration details

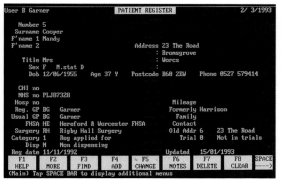

Registration details.

All systems record comprehensive demographic details about every patient registered with the practice (permanent and temporary) and have an archive of information about those who have left. When the practice is first computerised basic details (name, address, date of birth, NHS number, registered general practitioner, etc) are normally transferred from the family health services authority computer on a tape. Subsequent maintenance of the database is the responsibility of the practice. New patients are usually added to the system by the receptionists as they register. Some practices are now able to transmit this registration data back to the family health services authority.

Once a basic record has been created the practice needs to summarise the old notes and put essential details such as recall dates for vaccinations or smear tests into the computer as soon as possible. Future systems may allow full electronic data interchange (EDI) between practices, which would save time and reduce the risk of transcription error.

## Adding data

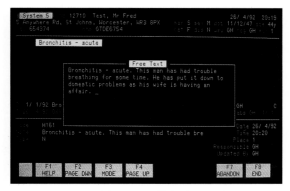

Adding a new problem to a clinical record.

Most practices now use their systems to record comprehensive details of every consultation. In addition to the date and time, the system records who saw the patient together with symptoms, signs, diagnoses, procedures carried out, and all drugs prescribed. Older systems recorded these details as text entries, but they are now automatically converted into (and stored as) Read codes. Some systems are limited to chronological recording in the form of a journal. Others use the familiar problem oriented approach in which all details about key problems such as ischaemic heart disease or malignancy are kept together so that it is easier to find and retrieve information about these problems later. Details about simple, unrelated problems (colds, sore throats, minor injuries, etc) can be put in a separate "pigeon hole" so that they do not clutter up the screen and obscure important problems. Good systems display a list of all serious problems as soon as a patient's record is retrieved.

## Creating computerised prescriptions

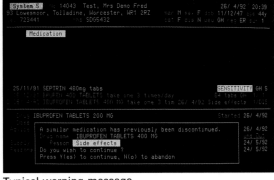

Typical warning message.

Computerised prescribing offers many advantages. Perhaps the most obvious is that prescriptions are always legible, greatly reducing the risk of dispensing errors. Since the prescriptions are all created from an accurate, regularly updated list of drugs and doses the risk of error is further reduced. Furthermore, when linked to the clinical record, new prescriptions are automatically cross referenced against current problems and medical history. Warnings of potential contraindications or a reminder that the drug has had to be discontinued in the past owing to allergy or intolerance further increase safety. Hand written prescriptions are still required, however, for controlled drugs.

# Clinical computer systems in general practice

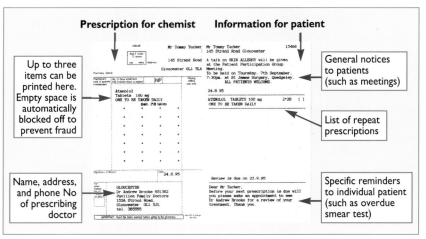

**Prescription for chemist** → **Information for patient**

Up to three items can be printed here. Empty space is automatically blocked off to prevent fraud

Name, address, and phone No of prescribing doctor

General notices to patients (such as meetings)

List of repeat prescriptions

Specific reminders to individual patient (such as overdue smear test)

Typical computer generated prescription (FP10Comp).

*Drug budget*

Management of the drug budget is also important. All systems can guide the prescriber towards a practice formulary but are flexible enough to allow exceptions to the rule when necessary. Accurate statistics on individual and group prescribing patterns help to contain costs. It is also easy to identify patients requiring expensive treatment (and therefore the conditions for which those drugs are being prescribed) should the practice be asked to justify its costs. The statistics are also invaluable for therapeutic audit.

## Creating reports

### Typical reports

Cervical cytology recall
Immunisation recall
Child health surveillance
Item of service claims
Referral data
Rural mileage
Clinical audits

Having invested so much time entering information about your practice, you will be in a good position to extract valuable information. The system can be instructed to search the database and return the answer to your question in the form of a report. Systems are usually supplied with most of the standard reports that a practice is likely to need. Producing a report is then as simple as selecting it from a menu. A report can take many forms—for example, a graph of activity for a business meeting or a list of patients due to have a cervical smear in the next month. Lists of patients can be merged with standard letters to produce a personalised letter to each patient on the list. Providing everyone has been diligent about entering accurate information, reports will reflect that accuracy. Such accuracy is much more difficult to achieve with a paper system and will help to ensure that government targets are met. Clinical reports allow you to search for all patients taking a specific drug (useful if there is a drug alert) or with a particular diagnosis such as diabetes or asthma.

## Appointments

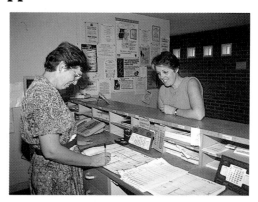

Use of traditional appointment book

Computerised appointment systems offer great flexibility in making and checking appointments but have to be extremely well written to be more usable than the traditional appointment book at the reception desk. One strength of the book is that it readily allows the receptionist an overview of activity in the practice, whereas computerised systems often show just one doctor's appointments at a time, making it more difficult to spot gaps where an urgent appointment could be fitted in.

Computerised systems do, however, have several useful advantages. Good systems automatically offer patients a choice of dates and times. Access to the appointment system is available at all terminals in a practice, and it is therefore possible for a doctor or practice nurse to make a follow up appointment before a patient leaves the consulting room. Making an appointment this way can be as simple as typing 2W or 3M (for two weeks or three months respectively). The system then searches for a vacant slot at about the right time. This relieves some of the pressure on receptionists, freeing time for other clerical tasks.

```
Appt  Consult  Edit  Find  General  HomeVisits  Joint  Move  Next  View  eXit
  APPTS for Dr Dennis            **BROWSE**              MONDAY 2/1/1995

Weekly Meeting                   10.40:.POLLY GRAHAM
                                         Immunisation 10 mins
                                 10.50:.RUSSELL WILLIAMS

                                 11.00:.MARION TANDY
  9.30:.                                 Extra 5 mins
                                 11.10:.BRIAN FELLOWSIingrowing toenail
  9.40:.HELEN SMITH(Joint)                Minor Op 30 mins
        Minor Op 30 mins


                                 11.40:.
10.10:.ELIZABETH BROWN
                                 11.50:.
10.20:.JOHN TELSON
        Blood test 10 mins       12.00:.
10.30:.
     F1=HELP  F2=ADD  F3=DELETE  F4=TRANSFER  F5=ARRIVED       <x> to EXIT
```

Computerised appointment system.

Most computerised systems automatically generate lists of patients to be seen by each doctor. During a consultation, the relevant list can be viewed on the doctor's terminal. Simply pointing to a name on the list calls up the patient's record, saving the time taken to search for it. Computerised systems also provide practices with statistics on consultation rates and workload and can be used to audit waiting times and to help practices to meet the targets set in the patient's charter.

# Writing referral letters

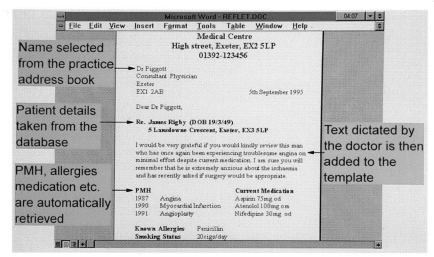

Name selected from the practice address book

Patient details taken from the database

PMH, allergies medication etc. are automatically retrieved

Text dictated by the doctor is then added to the template

Creating a referral letter from computer database. These same details can be passed automatically to fundholding software for future reconciliation with an invoice from the hospital.

General practitioners write many referral letters each week, making a great deal of work for a practice secretary. Good letters contain details of a patient's medical history, current problems, and any drugs being taken. All of these details are held in the database and can therefore be retrieved for use in referral letters—saving the trouble of typing them out each time. Furthermore, you can create an address book containing details of the hospitals, clinics, and consultants to whom your practice's patients are commonly referred. Most systems include a basic word processor linked to the database and a series of customisable letter templates.

To create a referral letter, the secretary picks an appropriate template selects the relevant consultant from the address book, and then merges both registration and clinical data from the patient's record into the template letter. Although this sounds complex, it can usually be done with just a few keystrokes. This saves time and reduces the risk of error in transcribing from a patient's notes. It is then a simple matter to type in the text dictated by the doctor.

At present letters are generally printed out and sent by post, but in future they are likely to be sent to their destination electronically via the NHS network.

# Online information

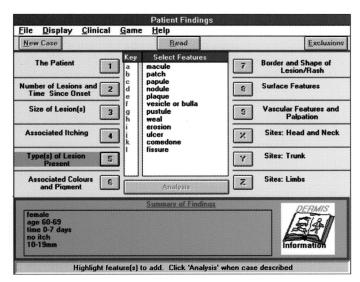

Programs such as this prototype expert system from EMIS provide invaluable help in reaching a diagnosis.

As general practice systems move over to the Windows environment, you will also be able to access colour photographs and diagrams or use networked CD ROMs. These will not only aid diagnosis but might also be useful to illustrate a point to your patients.

Given the ever expanding knowledge base in medicine it is impossible for a doctor to have expertise in all areas. In recognition of this many general practice systems now include a variety of online resources. These usually allow you to call up specific information about a particular disease or drug, but systems which analyse symptoms and signs and suggest appropriate investigations or a differential diagnosis are being developed.

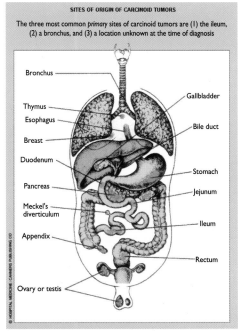

SITES OF ORIGIN OF CARCINOID TUMORS

The three most common *primary* sites of carcinoid tumors are (1) the ileum, (2) a bronchus, and (3) a location unknown at the time of diagnosis

The Merck Manual on CD ROM allows easy access to comprehensive information on a wide variety of topics

# Developments in general practice computing

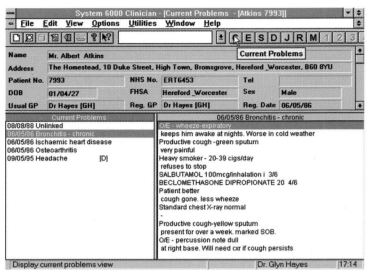

Meditel's new System 6000.

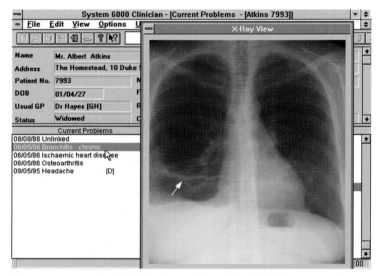

Future systems will include advanced graphical displays.

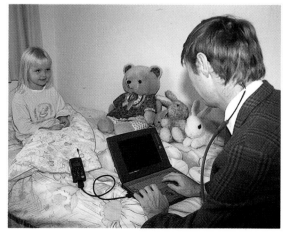

Using a portable computer during a home visit.

## Upgrading software

In common with a general move away from character based interfaces to the modern graphical user interface, the next generation of general practice software has been designed to run on Windows based computers. The screens are much more attractive for doctors and patients to look at, and the increasingly familiar Windows interface is far more intuitive to use, reducing the time needed for staff training.

A further advantage is the ability to run these new general practice programs alongside other standard Windows software and to transfer information easily from one to the other. The ability to record and display simple graphics such as line drawings will enhance clinical records. In the future it may also be possible to download $x$ rays over the NHS network, and these can be stored and displayed alongside other patient information as shown.

## Upgrading hardware

Current systems using dumb terminals are unable to run Windows. To be able to use the newer systems, practices will need to invest in a lot of new hardware. For example, each of the terminals will need to be upgraded to a modern PC. Current wiring systems with serial cables limit the speed at which information can be moved around a practice, and this is one reason for the sluggish response of today's computers. These serial cables will also need to be replaced by modern fast network wiring. Many suppliers are already installing such networks in all new installations.

## Portable computing

At present, very few practices have the facility to take a computer on home visits, but this option is attractive, particularly in large practices where patients are not well known to each partner. Entering details of a consultation at the time would also avoid the need to return to the practice to record the visit. It is possible to transfer the patient database on to a portable computer at the end of each day and to take that computer with you while on call, but it is then necessary to lock all the records on the computer at the practice until any changes made on the portable computer have been transferred back on to the main system. Failure to do this might jeopardise the integrity of the database. However, the recent development of digital mobile phones, such as Orange or GSM, and notebook computers has raised the possibility of dialling into the main practice computer wherever you are—at your house, on home visits, or even while out and about in your car. The move to Windows 95 will make this kind of remote computing much easier to set up.

| Major suppliers of general practice computer systems | |
|---|---|
| *Company* | *Telephone No.* |
| AAH Meditel | 01527 579414 |
| EMIS | 0113 259 1122 |
| VAMP Health | 0171 498 1330 |
| GPASS (Scotland) | 0141 882 9996 |

Fortunately, these major system upgrades can be done gradually over several years, and practices can use a mixture of old and new hardware in the intervening period. At present, many practices are likely to decide not to increase their investment in their computer system. However, practices planning to move to new premises or to purchase a new system may choose to take advantage of the benefits of these new systems straight away. In time, all systems become obsolete, and you will need to make financial allowance for upgrading both hardware and software.

# 16 MANAGING GP COMPUTER SYSTEMS

## Support

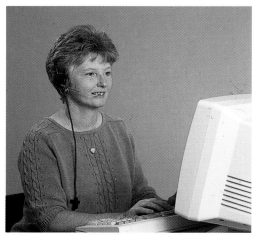

Computer help desks provide easy access to expert advice.

*Service contracts*

Computer systems are generally very reliable, but both hardware and software sometimes fail. Practices that are dependent on a computer to perform key tasks are vulnerable to considerable disruption if the system crashes. It is therefore essential that the practice has a maintenance contract with the supplier of the system and easy access to a help desk during normal surgery hours. Many crashes are not due to equipment failure but occur because of operator error. Fortunately, many of these problems are relatively simple to sort out in a few minutes given clear advice over the telephone. More complex problems are best resolved by the supplier using a modem and remote control software. This allows the supplier to take control of the system to fix the problem, after which it is returned to your control.

Hardware failures are more of a problem, and it is usually necessary to call out an engineer to repair the fault. It is sometimes possible to avoid call outs and reduce maintenance costs by keeping a few simple spares in stock. Dumb terminals, for example, can be replaced easily without special knowledge. The maintenance contract should stipulate the maximum call out time—preferably no more than eight hours. Before committing to a particular computer system, practices should consult existing users to ascertain the effectiveness of the support offered to them in past crises.

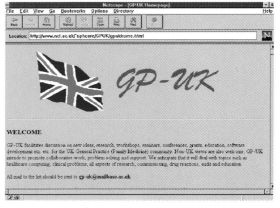

GP-UK Internet home page.

*User groups*

In addition to support from the supplier, colleagues who have long experience of using the system are often able to answer common questions and may well have found a way around apparent limitations in the software. It is therefore worthwhile finding out if there is a user group in your area. Most run regular, well supported meetings. In addition to problem solving and disseminating information about future developments, these groups provide valuable feedback to suppliers. Information gained from users can be used to track down and resolve bugs in the software and stimulates development of new features in response to popular demand.

Some user groups run bulletin board systems (BBS), allowing anyone to dial in, read the latest news, post messages and questions, and retrieve answers. The national bulletin boards provide a means of making contact with distant colleagues who share similar interests and are well worth exploring. The Internet opens up new possibilities. The Primary Healthcare Specialist Group of the British Computer Society and the Sowerby Unit at Newcastle University both run a series of world wide web pages containing a wealth of information about new developments. Similarly, the major software companies have created well illustrated web sites describing their programs in great detail. These pages are available to primary care physicians anywhere in the world.

# Training

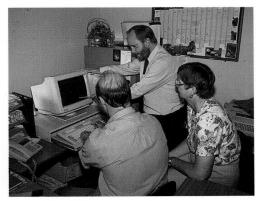

Training session.

Training goes hand in hand with support. It is essential to set aside time for effective training in order to maximise the return on your investment. Suppliers of new systems are usually keen to provide training as soon as possible after installation as this reduces the workload on their help desk. It is most cost effective for key members of staff to receive this expert training first. When they have mastered the system their skills can be cascaded through a practice at little expense. New staff merit particular attention, and everyone should have a periodic update as computer systems tend to evolve slowly. Failure to address this important issue leaves a practice vulnerable to errors and financial loss.

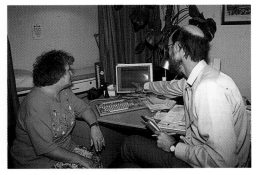

Using computer in consulting room.

*Positioning the computer screen*

It is also worth devoting some time to other important factors such as the way people interact with a computer while dealing with a patient. Staff should be taught to be careful not to leave confidential data on screen where it might be seen by other patients. At reception it is therefore best to have the screen facing away from the counter. In the privacy of the consulting room, however, you might wish to be able to share information on screen with a patient in order to foster trust and to reinforce your advice. Turning away from the patient to face the computer is far from ideal as this breaks the continuity of the consultation and leaves the patient staring at your back. The photograph shows an ideal arrangement.

# Security

### Choosing a password

- Use minimum of six characters
- Avoid obvious names (such as those of children or pets)
- Avoid complex combinations (such as "GTFAZRQS")
- Consider using two common but unconnected words separated by a typographic symbol: "tree/dog", "grass@chair", or "money#water"
- Never share your password
- Change your password regularly

*Passwords*

Passwords are the standard way of restricting access to most computer systems and are essential if the system is to meet official standards. In addition to controlling general access to the system, passwords can be used to restrict access selectively to sensitive parts of the database (such as staff records) and to limit users' options. Thus, receptionists can be authorised to issue repeat prescriptions but prevented from creating new ones. Furthermore, there are certain maintenance functions which, if used incorrectly, could be very damaging. Access to these should be limited to the system supervisor (usually the practice manager or the partner with responsibility for the computer system), who will have had special training to use them properly. Every member of staff is allocated a unique password by the system manager. These should never be shared or written down. If a password is compromised, it should be cancelled immediately and a new one issued.

**The best way to protect a system is by educating staff to the danger.**

*Viruses*

General practice systems are not invulnerable to computer viruses, but until recently the risk has been low because most common viruses do not infect the kind of operating system used in general practice computers. However, as new Windows based systems become more widely used, the risk will increase. Most viruses are transmitted on floppy disks, and, as the floppy disk drive is not needed once the software has been installed, disabling the drive is an excellent defence. You may, however, need help from the supplier to do this. Going on line to a bulletin board system poses a small threat—but only if programs are downloaded and run before being checked with a virus scanner.

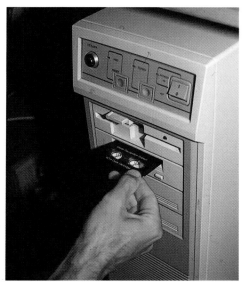

Tape streamer.

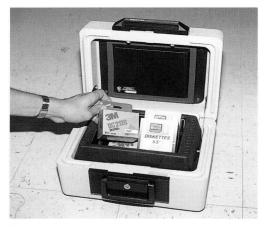

Fireproof data safe.

*Backups*

The information held on a practice computer is the most valuable part of the system and is often irreplaceable. When faults occur the database sometimes becomes corrupted, and it is impossible to get the system up and running reliably. It is therefore vitally important that a practice strictly follows a regular backup routine so that a recent copy is always available in the event of an emergency. Once any faults have been repaired, the supplier will restore data back onto the system from the most recent backup. Most current systems use a tape streamer to transfer data from the hard disk onto a tape cartridge. You should buy several tapes, regularly rotate them, and replace them annually as they tend to wear out. Backups should be taken at least once a day—more often if the system is used heavily. Some systems require that all users log off before running the backup. This can be disruptive, but it may be possible to automate the process so that it runs during a quiet period —for example, at lunchtime or overnight. You should also maintain a written log of every backup.

Never store backup tapes beside the computer as they would then be just as vulnerable to fire or theft as the computer. The best policy is to store most of the tapes in a fireproof data safe, but at least one copy should always be kept in a secure place somewhere off the premises.

# Medicolegal considerations

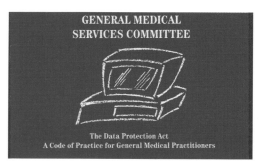

The BMA and medical defence organisations provide useful booklets on medicolegal issues.

In addition to the statutory requirement to comply with the Data Protection Act and the Display Screen Equipment Regulations, there are several specific medicolegal issues to consider when using a computer system. The current terms of service stipulate that general practitioners must record details of every consultation and prescription on paper as well as on the computer. This duplication of records is inefficient, and the government is currently looking at ways to legitimise the electronic record. Development of secure audit trails, which create an indelible chronological log of each action, will greatly ease many concerns and will be an important step along the road towards the paperless practice. At present, the medical defence organisations prefer paper records as the validity of electronic records has not yet been fully tested in the courts.

# Requirements for accreditation (RFA)

The Department of Health has stipulated that, in order to qualify for the reimbursement scheme, computer systems must offer the following features (among others)
- Use of the new NHS number
- Recording of certain key details:
    Clinical information
    Call and recall dates
    Item of service claims
- Read codes
- A secure audit trail
- Secure access control (passwords)
- Telephone support by supplier
- Electronic Data Interchange (EDI)
- Links to local family health services authority (registration and item of service)
- ESCROW agreement

*Requirements for accreditation*

The Department of Health has developed a set of minimum standards which general practice computing systems must meet if they are to qualify for reimbursement. It is likely that some suppliers will be unable to make the necessary changes to their systems and that this will result in mergers and therefore a smaller number of larger suppliers. One of the most important requirements is the establishment of an ESCROW agreement, in which the source code for the software is deposited with a third party on the understanding that it will be released to users of the system if the supplier goes out of business or withdraws from the market. This agreement is essential in order to protect users' investment in the system, which would otherwise be lost.

# Electronic links

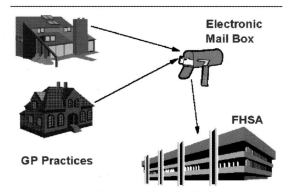

General practice links with local family health services authority.

*EDIFACT (Electronic Data Interchange For Administration Commerce and Transport)* is a European standard which has been adopted by the NHS. Once it has been incorporated into all health care computer systems it will allow data to be seamlessly transferred between them. It already underpins general practices' links to family health services authorities and hospital pathology systems and is likely to form the basis for the new NHS-wide network. The links project offers the opportunity for practices to exchange data electronically with their local family health services authority. The practice computer and that of the family health services authority are not directly linked together; rather information is left in an electronic mailbox to be collected by the other computer at a convenient time. This makes the practice computer secure against unauthorised use. Initially the system is limited to the transfer of registration data—details about patients joining or leaving a practice. Later, item of service (IOS) claims may be submitted electronically, enabling a practice to claim for work done without having to complete a separate claim form for each procedure. The system is policed by a system of retrospective audit. Practices may also link up with hospital laboratories to collect results of tests the moment they have been completed.

# 17   COMPUTERISING THE BUSINESS SIDE OF GENERAL PRACTICE

## Administration

**Business applications used in general practice**

- Word processor
- Payroll program
- Spreadsheet
- Accounts package
- Fundholding software
- Online banking
- Desktop publishing

Many modern practice computer systems are equipped with a separate PC on which the practice manager can run various standard business programs. These workstations can be connected to the main system by using terminal emulation software that makes them behave like dumb terminals. This allows the practice manager to access the patient database as well. Good systems allow the manager to transfer data from the clinical system into the business programs for further analysis of activity and profitability. Many practices choose to put a laser printer in the practice manager's office so that professional looking letters, reports, notices, and leaflets can be produced.

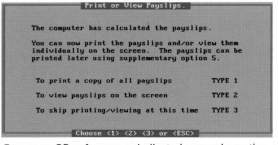

Ferguson GP software: a dedicated general practice payroll system.

### Managing the payroll

All practice managers will be familiar with the problems of using paper based payroll systems. Tax and national insurance deductions have to be looked up in the correct tables, payslips have to be written out by hand, and returns to the inland revenue have to be calculated manually. The process is particularly laborious when a practice has more than about 10 employees and is liable to simple arithmetic errors.

Computerised payroll systems greatly simplify the whole process and ensure a high degree of accuracy. In addition to automatically calculating tax and national insurance deductions, they are all capable of handling statutory sick pay and maternity leave payments. Furthermore, they print out tax returns approved by the inland revenue—P60s at the end of the year and P45s when employees leave. There are several excellent commercial systems, but practice managers often prefer to use systems written specifically for general practice (such as the Ferguson system) because they also produce the quarterly returns required by family health services authorities to calculate reimbursement of staff salaries.

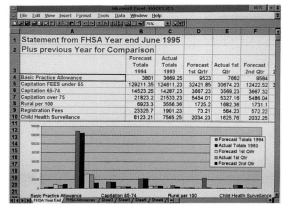

Using a spreadsheet to monitor cashflow.

### Monitoring cash flow

All practices must closely monitor their income and outgoings to ensure that optimal cash flow is maintained. This task is not easy given the very complex mixture of income from a wide variety of sources and both regular and irregular expenses. To make the task more difficult, payments from family health services authorities to general practices are uneven, with large quarterly sums and smaller interim monthly adjustments.

A spreadsheet can be programmed to monitor this complex situation so that the current and projected balance in a practice's bank accounts can be instantly calculated at any time. Results are normally printed in the form of a table but can readily be converted into a graph for easy viewing. Spreadsheets also allow the manager to consider the effect of different business plans such as taking on a new partner or dropping one type of work in favour of another. The manager and partners are then able to make informed decisions about whether a new venture would be financially viable.

## Useful accounts and payroll programs

|  | Telephone No |
|---|---|
| QuickBooks | 0500 585058 |
| Tass Books | 0181 874 6511 |
| Pegasus | 01536 518000 |
| Sage product range | 0191 255 3000 |
| Ferguson Payroll | 0831 387068 |
| McLean Accounts | 0141 616 0691 |
| Freeway Payroll (Shareware) | 01892 663298 |

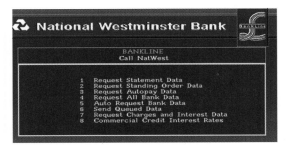

A modern, easy to use accounts package.

### Bookkeeping

It is essential to maintain a complete record of a practice's financial activities so that accurate accounts can be drawn up by the practice's accountant at the end of the year. Traditionally, all financial transactions are recorded in a paper based, double entry bookkeeping system—a complex but well established way of keeping track of money as it flows in and out of a practice's accounts. Some practices use a much simpler cashbook system, in which a chronological log of all income and outgoings are recorded. The entries in the book (ledger) are regularly checked against other records such as invoices or bank statements—a process known as reconciliation.

A computerised ledger is ideal for this task as the calculations involved can be performed extremely quickly and accurately. Furthermore, reports generated by these programs reduce the time taken to produce the annual accounts, with a corresponding reduction in the cost of accountancy. You should seek your accountant's advice before committing to a particular program to ensure that it is suitable on financial grounds and that it is compatible with the software used by the accountancy firm.

### Fundholding

The sheer complexity of managing a fundholding practice makes computerisation essential. Special fundholding software has been developed by most of the large computer system suppliers. These must conform to a series of rigid standards laid down by the Department of Health in order to qualify for accreditation. Reimbursement is available only for systems that meet these standards.

Typical fundholding system. Fully integrated programs that automatically pass referral data from the clinical database into the fundholding system reduce the need to duplicate entry of data.

These fundholding systems can be fully integrated with a practice's clinical system or can operate independently from it, but all are required to analyse activity and produce reports in a standard format. This simplifies NHS administration and allows easy comparison of financial and administrative data between practices and geographical areas.

Unlike non-fundholding practices, which are entitled to receive a maximum of 50% reimbursement providing that the family health services authority has sufficient money available, fundholding practices can currently deduct up to 75% of the cost of additional hardware required to run the fundholding program from their management allowance.

### Electronic (online) banking

Practices equipped with a PC and modem can subscribe to the 24 hour online banking services offered by several banks. Access to the service is strictly controlled through the use of passwords known only to the practice, ensuring both privacy and security. Use of these services allows a practice's partners or practice manager access to information about every aspect of the practice's accounts, including recent credits or debits and the current balance. It also allows them to transfer funds between accounts and to pay bills or staff salaries, order statements, and leave email messages for the bank. Data obtained from the system can be transferred into a standard spreadsheet for further financial analysis. Bank charges are often much reduced if transactions are carried out on line, but the savings need to be carefully balanced against the cost of subscribing to the service.

Some banks offer comprehensive online services.

## Desktop publishing

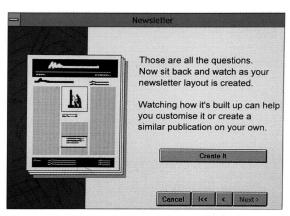

It is easy to create effective posters and leaflets.

While it is possible to use a modern word processor to design notices, leaflets, and reports, there are several user friendly desktop publishing programs that allow you to create interesting and effective layouts without special knowledge. These programs use "handholding" techniques to guide you through the process one step at a time, and it is possible to produce professional looking documents in just a few minutes. After they are saved to the hard disk, they can easily be updated and reused at any time in the future. Many practices use desktop publishing to produce their annual report, a regular newsletter, or series of patient information leaflets.

# 18 NETWORKS AND HOSPITAL BASED COMPUTER SYSTEMS

A computer's usefulness is greatly enhanced if it is connected to others in a network, as this allows information and resources to be shared by all. A network can be anything from a simple link between two computers in an office to a complex installation joining thousands of computers at many sites around the world.

In a hospital two types of networks are commonly found. The first is the local area network (LAN), which is typically used to connect the secretaries and medical staff in one department. This allows everyone to use and build up a departmental database and to use standard letter templates for correspondence (such as clinic letters and discharge summaries), which saves time and greatly facilitates audit and research.

The second type is the wide area network (WAN), such as a hospital-wide system that connects all departments to a central computer running a patient administration system (PAS) with microwave or leased line links to outlying hospitals and clinics. Such networks are primarily designed to manage hospital activity (such as outpatient appointments, theatre lists, etc). Information about hospital activity extracted from these systems is required by purchasers and the Department of Health.

---

**Advantages of networking**

- Sharing of data and programs
- Sharing of computer peripherals (such as printers, modems, CD ROMs
- Security
- Email and faxing
- Allows access to network via a telephone line
- Cost effectiveness

---

## Departmental networks

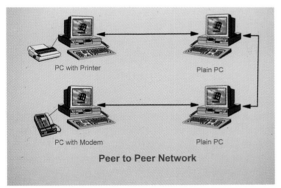

Peer to Peer Network

Peer to peer network: all users can share each other's work and resources.

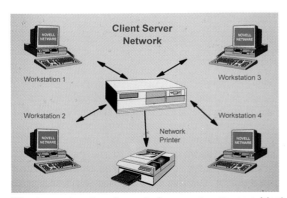

Client server network: central computer stores critical data and programs

### Peer to peer networks

This is the simplest type of network and is ideal for linking a small number of computers together. The key feature of a peer to peer network is that all computers connected to it can be considered equal. Any hardware attached to one computer—such as a printer, CD ROM drive, or fax modem—can be made available to all computers on the network. Furthermore, users can, if they wish, easily share data stored on their hard discs with their colleagues. Peer to peer networks are very easy to set up, requiring only a network card in each computer and network cable to join them together. If you are setting up a peer to peer network with modern computers, Windows for workgroups and Windows 95 both contain all the software that you need. If you are using older computers incapable of running Windows you will need DOS based software such as LANtastic or Novell Personal Netware.

### Client server networks

For systems in which security is important (such as clinical systems) the client server network is a much better choice. Here, all the data (and programs if necessary) are held on a central computer called a file server to which all the other computers, called workstations, are connected. The advantage of this arrangement is that the file server can be locked away in a secure room, protected from physical risks such as fire or theft.

Furthermore, access to data and programs can be strictly controlled by means of separate passwords assigned to each user. Programs (such as word processors or databases) can be set up so that files are automatically saved on the file server, making the network appear totally transparent to the user. Backing up the file server is much easier and quicker than it would be if data were stored on several different workstations.

When setting up any type of departmental network in a hospital you should seek advice and support from the hospital computer department

File servers make extensive use of temporary memory (RAM), which greatly speeds up busy networks, but they are therefore vulnerable to failure of mains power and consequential loss of data. To safeguard against this, all file servers should be connected to an uninterruptable power supply (UPS) unit containing a rechargeable battery that keeps the file server going in the event of a mains power failure. Meanwhile, special software copies any unsaved data to the hard disc before automatically closing down the network.

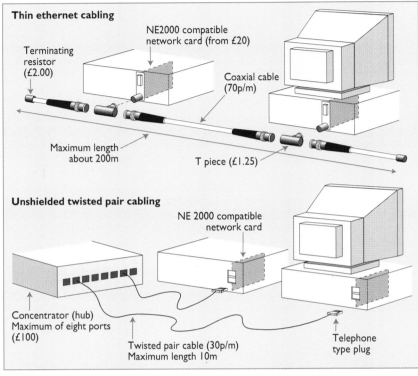

Network cabling: thin ethernet and unshielded twisted pair (UTP).

*Network cabling*

*Thin ethernet*—The simplest and cheapest cabling system is thin ethernet, which uses coaxial cable to loop from one computer to the next in a daisy chain up to about 200 m long. Each computer is connected to the chain with a T piece, and each end of the chain must be terminated with a special plug containing a resistor. The cables and connectors must be protected from physical damage as any break in the chain will cause the whole network to fail (crash).

*Unshielded twisted pair (UTP)* cabling is far more robust as damage to a cable will result in only one computer dropping out of the network. Furthermore, each computer is connected to the hub with a single telephone like cable, which is a much tidier arrangement.

*Large networks* linking several floors in a building or a number of different buildings use thick ethernet, token ring, or fibre optic cables. The latter operates 10 times faster and can carry much more traffic than standard cabling systems and is therefore ideal for large hospitals.

# Hospital networks

### Features of a hospital patient administration system

*Clinics*—Managing patient attendance, sending appointment letters
*Wards*—Patient admission and discharge, bed occupancy
*Pathology services*—From requests to results
*Operating theatres*—Theatre lists, reporting of operations actually carried out
*Reports of hospital activity*

*Patient administration system*

The patient administration system is a generic name for the computer software that looks after the administrative aspects of patient care. At its core is a large database containing basic details (such as name, address, telephone number, general practitioner, and hospital number) about all of the hospital's patients. Historically, the patient administration system was used primarily to record details of admissions and outpatient appointments, but it has evolved considerably and is now linked to a wide variety of departments and records and supports many key activities.

*Appointments systems*

One of the advantages of a centralised system is that appointments can be made not only by clinic receptionists and the medical records department but also by a ward nurse before a patient is discharged and by a consultant's secretary in response to an urgent request from a general practitioner. When an appointment is made or changed the system can automatically send an appropriate letter to the patient. In advance of each clinic, lists of the names of patients due to attend can be printed out and can then used by the medical records department to retrieve the correct notes. Comprehensive information about past and future appointments can be analysed for planning purposes.

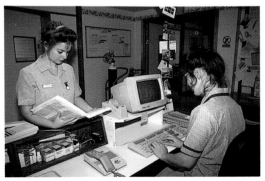

Ward nurses can make appointments on a centralised computer system.

```
                PAS - Pathology Request Form
CRN      P894532k   Order No 1      Date 29/8/95  10/01
Name     John Soap  Sex   Male      DOB 12/3/45
Location  Paget Ward                Consultant G. Smith

01  Details    Patient clinical anaemic

02  Exam required [........]    Press F2/f7 for Help
07  Urgency        [...]      08  Transport [...]
09  Date required  [........]
10  Pt IP/OP       [...]
11  Date of LMP    [...]       12  Ignore LMP [...]
14  Allergies      [......................]
15  Drugs          [......................]
```

Computerised pathology request form.

## Some of the reports NHS hospitals have to generate

*Korner reports*
Such as
   KH06—Information about elective
     admissions
   MA02—Information about hospital waiting
     lists
   KH09—Information about consultant
     outpatient clinic activity
   KC61—Information about cervical cytology
     results
*Patient's charter returns*—Used to monitor standards set out in the patient's charter
*Hospital episode statistics (HES)*—Reports actual number of admissions
*Northern flat file (NFF)*
   Patient's address, details of general
     practitioner
   Consultant and specialty code
   Procedure coding
   Attendance date, clinic number
*Hospital activity matrix*—Sent monthly to health authority

## Electronic communication in the NHS

- General practitioners and hospitals for referrals, discharges, pathology results, outpatient appointments
- General practitioners and family health services authorities for registration details, items of service claims
- NHS local and central registers for changes in patient registration
- Family health services authorities' computer units for maintenance of systems and software
- Purchaser-provider links for reporting of hospital acitivity
- Family health service authorities and electronic prescription pricing and cost information (EPACT)
- NHS supplies and other NHS organisations for orders and invoicing
- Dentists and Dental Practice Board for claim for payments
- Email

## Pathology systems

Pathology departments were among the first to link their computers to the patient administration system, and in some hospitals results have been available over the network for several years. An increasing number of hospitals' systems now allow you to make pathology requests this way as well, with the advantage that requests are always legible and contain all the information that the laboratory needs. Paper records are still required for patients' notes, and some clinical departments and wards have a printer set up to automatically print out pathology results as soon as they are available.

## Department of Health returns

Hospital and community trusts are required to produce monthly reports on their activity. The best known of these are the Korner reports. There are currently over 65 of these for use by the Department of Health, covering key aspects of activity). In addition, hospitals are required to generate an electronic record of their inpatient activity (including ICD10 codes) called the northern flat file (NFF). This is sent to the regional computer centre, where it is sorted and analysed. The results are made available to purchasing authorities and general practitioner fundholders, who use it to pay hospitals for the work that they have done and to plan future purchasing strategies.

Much of the information for these reports is extracted from the patient administration system. It is therefore important that clinicians are aware of the data that is being collected from their department. Failure to accurately code and record all departmental activity on the computer system can result in loss of revenue to the hospital and may lead to inaccurate statistics about the work you have done.

## Connecting to other parts of the NHS

In response to general practitioners' demands for faster communication from hospitals (particularly after a patient's discharge), hospitals are exploring ways of communicating with them electronically. The simplest method, currently used by several hospitals, is to automatically generate a simple discharge summary as a patient leaves the hospital. This contains important clinical information such as diagnosis, treatment, and arrangements for follow up and is sent directly from the patient administration system to a secure fax machine at the surgery, thus minimising delays.

In the future this information is likely to be transferred directly into general practice computer systems via the new NHS-wide network. At present, links between hospital and general practice computer systems are limited, but pathology results are already being sent to suitably equipped practices.

## Training and passwords

Patient administration systems are now fundamentally important to the smooth running of hospitals, and all staff, including junior doctors, need to know how to use them. It is therefore essential to set aside time for training when new staff join an organisation. Passwords are the main way of restricting access to the confidential patient information held on hospital computers, and most hospitals will not issue passwords to staff until they have undergone training. In order to increase security, it is common practice for passwords to be changed periodically. Choosing and remembering a password can be difficult, but avoid using common words or names that could easily be associated with yourself. Select an unusual word at least six characters long, and consider adding unusual characters (£, $, %, @) to the word. Passwords should never be written down or shared with others.

# Paperless record systems

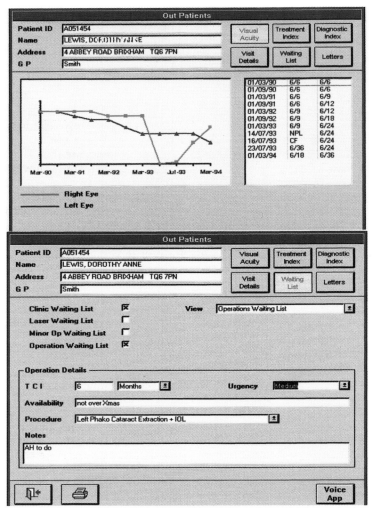

Screen shots of OphthBase: a paperless record system for ophthalmology departments.

General practices and many commercial organisations such as insurance companies have been working towards paperless systems for some years, but they are only just starting to emerge in hospitals. Patients' records are not only bulky but are often a disorganised collection of illegible handwritten notes, results, and correspondence that is all too commonly mislaid.

Computerised clinical record systems solve many of these problems. They have the additional advantage that any particular record can be accessed simultaneously in several different places; thus, a secretary can get on with typing a letter while the patient is being seen by a doctor elsewhere. Small scale, departmental systems already exist, but the main reasons why these systems are not yet common throughout hospitals are their complexity and cost.

Current systems use pick lists wherever possible to minimise the need to enter free text, but once recent advances in speech recognition have been fully exploited they will become even easier to use. Future systems will also probably include digitised electrocardiograms, x ray pictures, angiograms, scans, photographs, and videos. For medicolegal reasons, current systems run alongside paper records, but in the future such systems will almost certainly replace traditional paper based hospital notes.

# Pocket computers in clinical practice

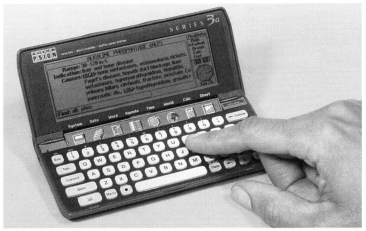

Palmtop computers can be used in clinical practice for storing reference values and calculating physiological data.

The screen shots of OphthBase were supplied by Palmtrees Medical Informatics, Torquay TQ1 2LN.

The increasing sophistication of palmtop computers is leading to their use in clinical practice. First generation palmtops were little more than electronic address books, but modern machines such as the Psion 3a are capable of many of the functions that would be expected of a PC. These include word processing, storing databases, scheduling appointments, and even sending faxes. They can also be connected to the main hospital network by mobile infrared or radio links – effectively a terminal in your pocket.

The ability to store large amounts of data (up to 10 Mb) makes palmtops ideal for storing reference material such as drug data (doses, trade names, interactions, side effects) and normal laboratory values. They can also help with tasks such as calculating rates of drug infusion or creatinine clearance and converting measurements to SI units (eg. mmHg to kPa).

# 19 ADAPTIVE COMPUTER TECHNOLOGY

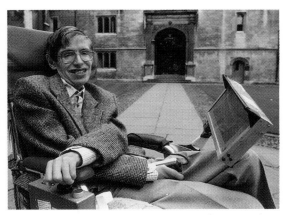

Professor Stephen Hawking uses adaptive computer technology to communicate.

People with a wide range of disabilities may be helped by adapting computer technology to suit their needs. In many cases, only relatively simple modifications are needed to allow disabled people to use standard computers at home or at work. In more severe cases computers can be adapted to allow disabled people who cannot move, see, or speak to communicate effectively.

For example, Professor Stephen Hawking, who has been severely disabled with motor neurone disease for many years, has written dozens of papers and a best selling book with the help of this type of technology. Furthermore, he lectures and regularly speaks on both radio and television programmes. To allow him to do this, his wheelchair has been fitted with a battery powered computer linked to a sensitive microswitch. Small hand movements are used to select words on a VDU screen mounted on the arm of his wheelchair. These words can be assembled into documents, which can be printed out later or can be fed into a speech synthesiser that reads and then speaks the phrases that he has created.

## Specialised hardware and software

### Conditions that may be helped by adaptive computer technology

*Sensory*
- Visual impairment  • Deafness

*Neurological*
- Cerebral palsy  • Dysphonia  • Dyslexia  • Head injury
- Multiple sclerosis  • Motor neurone disease  • Tremor  • Stroke

*Other*
- Deformity or injury to hands or arms
- Work related upper limb disorder (WRULD)

Special hardware and software are now available that can accommodate most disabilities and allow disabled people to use all the functions of a computer. It is no longer necessary for the user to sit upright in front of a screen or even to be able to read a screen. Keyboards can be modified or replaced altogether with speech recognition technology. The now familiar mouse, which is extensively used in graphical user interfaces such as Windows, can be replaced by a tracker ball, light pen, or by a touch sensitive VDU screen. People with dyslexia are greatly helped by automatic spell checking. Much of this equipment is readily available at a reasonable price and is sometimes useful to able bodied people.

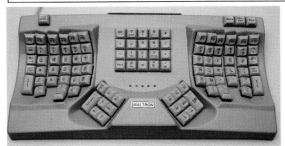

Keyboard designed to fit the hands and reduce muscular fatigue.

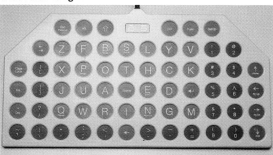

Keyboard with very large, easy to use keys.

### Special keyboards

Information is usually fed into a computer by means of a keyboard. Keyboards can be bought in a variety of shapes and sizes: some have been designed to avoid problems of muscular fatigue by having the keys arranged to fit the hands and with the most commonly used keys adjacent to different fingers. This contrasts with the standard "QWERTY" keyboard, which is designed for touch typists and requires the muscles of the hands and forearms to be in a state of constant static load above the keys. A simple wrist rest placed in front of a standard keyboard may help to reduce upper limb fatigue.

Small keyboards that can be accommodated in the lap are available, and even smaller ones, with the most commonly used keys in the centre, can be attached to the arm of a wheelchair for use by someone with very little arm movement. By contrast, keyboards with extra large keys may be useful for people without fine finger movements or who type with their toes.

# Adaptive computer technology

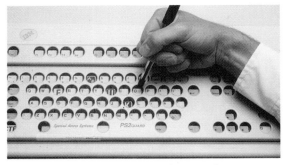

Standard keyboard fitted with a keyguard.

A keyguard lies over a keyboard and has holes above each key so that the user can rest the weight of his or her upper body on the keyboard while selecting and pressing keys. Keyguards are made of metal or rigid plastic and will fit most normal keyboards. Software is available to modify the keyboard response for someone who dwells too long on each keystroke or who cannot hit two keys simultaneously. Braille keyboards are available for use either in conjunction with or instead of a standard keyboard with IBM compatible computers.

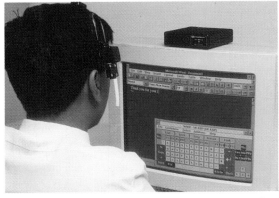

Keyboard emulation by means of head pointer and keyboard displayed on the screen.

## Keyboard emulation

People who are unable to use a keyboard can enter commands into the computer with devices such as a switch, mouse, tracker ball, joystick, or head pointer. These are used with a keyboard that is displayed on the computer screen; the required key is activated when it is highlighted by the input device. This is known as keyboard emulation. Because such a method of inputting is slower than using a keyboard it is often used in conjunction with "predictive software", which saves time by predicting the word or phrase that the user wants on the basis of the first few letters or words. The required word is then selected by a keystroke or emulation.

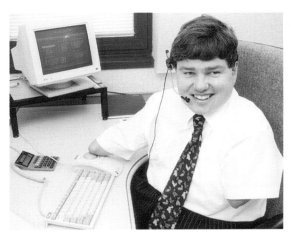

Solicitor with congenital limb deformities uses a tracker ball, small keyboard, and voice input to control his computer.

## Speech recognition

Speech recognition is available for people with conditions that prevent them from using a keyboard as well as for able bodied people who do not have typing skills or who need to keep their hands free during dictation. These systems work by recognising the phonemes that make up the spoken word. These are compared with an individual user's voice pattern and an electronic dictionary containing up to 120 000 words. Complex language analysis is used to distinguish between different words which sound the same—such as "to", "too", and "two". The software is also capable of deciding when "2" would be more appropriate (such as in a spreadsheet). Once the software has been "trained" to recognise the user's voice, speeds of up to 100 words a minute can be reached. Modern speech recognition software achieves an uncanny degree of accuracy and has the ability to learn from mistakes to become even more accurate with increasing use. Current systems require the user to dictate in isolated speech with a small gap between each word but systems that accurately recognise continuous speech are not far away.

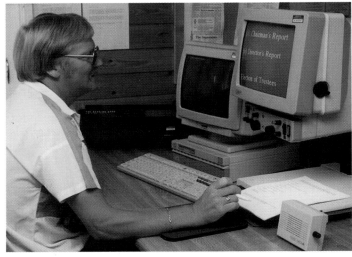

Partially sighted man using closed circuit television, conventional keyboard, speech synthesiser, and electronic reading machine.

## Adapting the screen

People with impaired vision may find that changing the colour of the text on the screen or the colour of the background can help, as can bringing the screen closer with an adjustable monitor arm. Large font software can be purchased, but this allows only a proportion of the original screen to be seen at any one time. A much better solution is to use large, high resolution monitors with a screen size of anything up to 33 inches, although these are very expensive. Standard text is then automatically enlarged. Many of these large monitors are best purchased through one of the mail order firms that advertise heavily discounted hardware in computer magazines. It would, however, be wise to choose a firm that will allow you to return the monitor if it proves unsuitable.

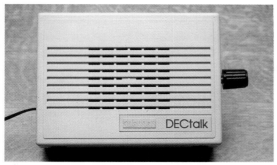

Simple speech synthesiser.

*Speech synthesisers*

If the user is unable to read any type of screen, special software can be used to "read" either the keys that are pressed or the contents of the screen. This information is then passed to a speech synthesiser. This is a device for producing intelligible speech by converting groups of letters into phonemes according to predetermined rules. Some voices may sound unnatural and the intonation poor, but they are rapidly improving in quality. This equipment may also be useful to people who cannot speak (like Professor Hawking), especially now that the voice can be adjusted to match the sex of the user.

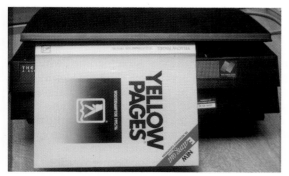

Electronic reading machine scanning page of telephone directory.

*Electronic reading*

Electronic reading machines convert printed text, such as the page of a book, into electronic speech or Braille output. These work by scanning the page to produce an electronic picture, which is then "read" by special optical character recognition (OCR) software. Accuracy depends on the type and quality of text printed on the page but, as with all technologies, it is improving very rapidly. Handwritten text cannot currently be recognised, but this can at least be enlarged and displayed for those who have some sight. Braille displays and embossers are also available, but since only a minority of visually impaired people can use Braille the market is small and they are relatively expensive.

# Choosing and buying equipment

## Sources of advice for disabled people

*ACE Centre*
Ormerod School, Waynflete Road, Headington, Oxford OX3 8DD
Telephone 01865 63508
Specialises in helping children with communication problems

*Blind in Business*
7 Rolls Buildings, Fetter Lane, London EC4A 1NH
Telephone 0171 931 5674
Charity that helps visually impaired people to find work

*Cambridge Adaptive Communication*
The Mount, Toft, Cambridge CB3 7RL
Telephone 01223 264244
Manufactures and supplies custom made equipment

*Computability Centre*
PO Box 94, Warwick CV34 5WS
Telephone 01926 312847
Charitable organisation that provides advice and personal assessments

*Dolphin Systems for People with Disabilities*
Unit 96C, Blackpole Trading Estate West, Worcester WR3 8TU
Telephone 01905 754577
Specialises in designing speech synthesisers and writing reading software

*Dragon Systems UK*
Pullar Close, Bishops Cleeve, Cheltenham GL52 4RW
Telephone 01242 678575
Produces Dragon Dictate speech recognition system

*Foundation for Communication for the Disabled*
25 High Street, Woking, Surrey GU21 1BW
Telephone 01483 727844

*Royal National Institute for the Blind*
224-226 Great Portland Street, London W1N 6AA
Telephone 0171 388 1266

*Sensory Systems*
1 Watling Gate, 297-303 Edgware Road, London NW9 6NB
Telephone 0181 205 3002
Supplies adaptive computer technology to visually impaired people

It is very important that anyone who is considering buying adaptive equipment should try it out before purchase in order to make sure that it will meet their needs. For people in work or planning to return to work, the Employment Service can spend up to £21 000 over five years to meet the cost of adaptive computer technology. Grants are also available for employers to adapt premises and to meet the cost of transport to and from work. The service has access to many companies specialising in this field and to independent experts who offer individual assessment of needs and unbiased advice. Help is also available for training and for job placements. For people not in work, there are limited loan and job introduction schemes. Any doctor or employer can refer disabled people to the service via the local disability employment adviser, who can be contacted at a Job Centre.

There is much that can be done for disabled people to help them realise their full potential. We may not be able to cure or treat the disability, but, thanks to modern electronics, we need no longer say, "There is nothing more I can do."

The authors thank Bill Fine of the Computability Centre and the Medical Illustration Department of Dudley Group Hospitals for their help. The photograph of Professor Hawking was supplied by Manni Masons Pictures, and the photograph of a solicitor with congenital limb deformities was supplied by Ernie Mitchell.

# 20   DIGITAL IMAGING

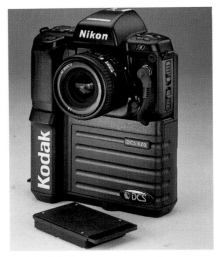

Kodak digital camera system based on Nikon F90 camera.

Traditionally pictures have been taken with photographic film, which then has to be processed before they can be viewed. The development of digital cameras now allows pictures to be taken and printed almost immediately. In medicine this can be an important advantage, and, even though the quality of digital images is currently lower than that of photographic film, the huge advantage of immediate images often far outweighs the slight loss of resolution. Digital cameras are now available to replace the standard 35 mm camera for taking routine clinical photographs as well as for use in specialised areas of medicine.

## Digital radiology

| Types of digital radiological imaging |
| --- |
| • Nuclear medicine |
| • Ultrasound |
| • Computed tomography |
| • Digital vascular imaging and digital subtraction angiograms |
| • Magnetic resonance imaging |
| • Digital fluorography |
| • Computed radiography |

Photographic film has served as the reception, storage, and display medium for x ray images for the past 100 years. Indeed, x rays were discovered because of their effect on photographic emulsion. When ultrasound scanning was developed the images were displayed on a monitor and were transitory. At that time digital storage was in its infancy, and it was impossible to store large numbers of images. Photographic film was cheap and readily available and so was chosen to provide a permanent record of the investigation.

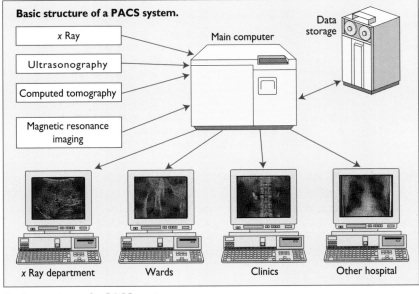

Basic structure of a PACS system.

However, with the current expansion in the variety of digitally acquired images and the increasing capacity of digital storage systems, the possibility of dispensing with photographic film has now arisen. Filmless imaging can lead to important savings in disposable resources and staff time and a major improvement in departmental efficiency.

*Picture archiving and communication system*

Storage of digital images is undertaken by a picture archiving and communication system (PACS). This term is now accepted jargon but, like all jargon, is becoming misused. Each component of PACS is fundamental to the success of the system. Pictures must be captured, stored, retrieved, distributed, and displayed at multiple sites for a system to be worthy of the name.

## Storage capacity needed to hold digital images

| Digital image | Size of image file |
|---|---|
| Ultrasound scan | 250 kb |
| Computed tomogram or magnetic resonance image | 1 Mb |
| Digital mammogram | 4 Mb |
| High resolution chest x ray | 16 Mb |
| One complete computed tomography or magnetic resonance imaging examination | 100 Mb |
| One week's digital images (uncompressed) | 100 000 Mb (100 gigabytes) |
| One year's digital images (uncompressed) | 5 000 000 Mb (5 terabytes) |
| One high density floppy disk | 1.4 Mb |
| Typical desk top PC hard disk | 800 Mb |

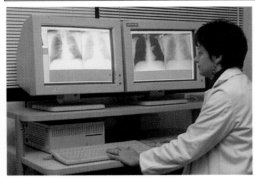

Workstation using two display screens for all types of radiological examinations.

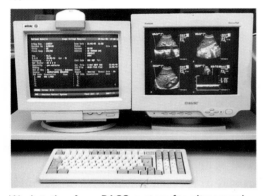

Workstation for a PACS system for ultrasound scans only, with one display screen and a patient data screen.

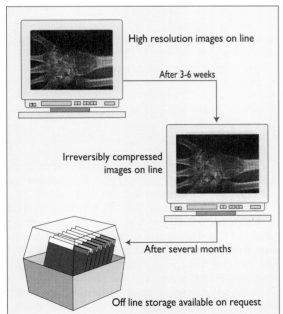

High resolution images on line

After 3-6 weeks

Irreversibly compressed images on line

After several months

Off line storage available on request

Sequence of image compression and storage.

Although this may seem simple, there are serious problems to be overcome. Almost all radiology systems produce their images in different formats, and the digital image files are often very large. Fortunately, the capacity of data storage systems is increasing at the rate of one order of magnitude every five years, and their costs are steadily reducing. However, the capacity required for a major radiology department to hold all its images permanently on line is still technologically and financially unachievable.

The display systems present a further obstacle. Radiologists are used to having eight or more viewing boxes of films on display at once, often with a mixture of examinations from one patient under review simultaneously. To reproduce this with large, high resolution computer screens and associated software is very expensive. Most practical systems use only two or four screens at each workstation. In addition the handling of electronic images requires very different disciplines from radiologists to those they are used to with film.

### Realistic systems

If a usable and cost effective system is to be implemented it is necessary to make a few compromises. The commonest options are:

*Store only certain examinations* (such as ultrasound, computed tomographic, or magnetic resonance scans). This has the advantage that the radiologist can get used to handling electronic images before being subjected to a totally digital environment, but the economies associated with lack of film will not be fully realised.

*Hold images on line for a limited period only*—This option is satisfactory if very few patients return for follow up examinations, but it can be a serious problem in a centre with many long term patients; exactly the type of institution that might benefit from PACS.

*Compress image data files*—This option is always practised to some degree. With modern software it is possible to compress an average radiology image file by about 2.5:1 with no loss of detail. Greater compression results in loss of data, so called "lossy" or "irreversible" compression. However, compressions of 6:1 are almost undetectable in the reconstructed image, and it has been claimed that a chest x ray can be compressed 25:1 before diagnostic information is lost.

In practice at least two of these options are followed in most digital departments to date. Most practical and effective PACS systems store all the department's images and have a "hot file" of rapidly accessible, "losslessly" compressed images that are less than a few weeks old. When an image has not been accessed for a period in excess of this it is irreversibly compressed and passed to the main archive. It can be retrieved from here more slowly. After a further period of inactivity, typically several months, images may be passed to an off line storage device and can be retrieved only when notice has been given in advance.

### Integration with management systems

Most large radiology departments now use computerised management systems. These systems hold all the details of patients' radiology history, appointments, reports, etc, and include a master index. If a PACS is added to such a system it is essential that the two are fully integrated. Surprisingly, this is often not done, and thus one may have to search for the images and the relevant report on two separate systems. Any new PACS system must include a fully functional departmental management system.

## Digital imaging

Brief clinical history (including Surgical Operations.) if relevant

*Known fibroids. growing bigger.
Please compare ;
previous loss of
16.11.94. Thanks*

PREGNANCY RULING

IGNORE ON GROUNDS OF URGENCY?
SIGNATURE OF DOCTOR:
..............................................

INFECTION RISK:     YES ☐     NO ☑
If YES, SPECIFY:

ARE YOU PREGNANT?
YES ☐     NO ☐

COULD YOU BE PREGNANT?

Part of a handwritten request form that had been scanned into a computer, compressed, and stored. It is then available for printing or display when required.

### Advantages of filmless imaging

- No film handling
- No film processing
- No enveloping of films
- No filing of film envelopes
- No retrieving of film envelopes
- No searching for lost films
- No sending films to wards or clinics
- Images rapidly available
- Greater efficiency
- Teleradiology

### Suppliers of digital imaging systems

| Company | Product | Telephone No |
| --- | --- | --- |
| Kodak | Digital camera system | 01753 830999 |
| Occulab | Digital fundus camera | 01753 857177 |
| ImageNet | Digital fundus camera | 01689 846700 |
| Philips | PACS system | 0181 741 1666 |
| Siemens | PACS system | 0181 740 3325 |
| SIMIS | PACS system | 01428 605055 |
| AMS | PACS system | 01296 696444 |

*Paperwork*—There is no logic in having a filmless department if paper request forms and reports still have to be handled and filed. Very few PACS systems address this problem. A fully functional radiology management and PACS system must include the facility for direct electronic requesting of examinations and should be able to convert paper requests into digital form for storage on the system. Only when this is achieved are the full advantages of a filmless and paperless department likely to be realised.

### Is PACS cost effective?

The capital cost of a full PACS system in a large hospital is currently likely to be of the order of tens of millions of pounds. The annual maintenance costs are likely to outweigh any possible staff savings from being filmless. The main gain will thus be in the speed, efficiency, and reliability of image retrieval from the archive and in communication. If a surgeon wants films in theatre all that is required is to call them up on the console; far quicker and more reliable than current x ray storage and retrieval services. Images can be available almost anywhere, even at a remote hospital if it is on the network (teleradiology). Computer technology has now just about reached the point when PACS becomes a realistic prospect for anyone designing a new department. It is not a cheap option, but in the new health service, where we are all more conscious of efficiency, it can allow us to offer a better service to our patients and colleagues.

### Data security

A filmless and paperless department will be totally incapacitated if the computer system breaks down. The record of PACS systems in Britain to date is not good in this respect. A well designed system must be capable of operating, even if only in crippled mode, during major failures of the power supplies or in the main components of the system. Ideally, all files should be duplicated, preferably by all the hard disks in the computer being duplicated, so called disk mirroring. This is technically possible but is financially unrealistic at present. Daily back up of all new data on to removable media, which are stored off site, is mandatory. If these rules are followed most catastrophes can be avoided.

## Digital ophthalmic photography

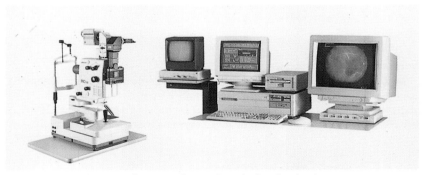

Computer based system for capturing and analysing fundus images.

Ophthalmologists use photographs to record retinal findings and to undertake fluorescein angiography. Traditionally, the film had to be processed, which meant that patients often had to return for a further clinic visit to get their results. Only Polaroid pictures are available instantly, but these are of rather low quality. The development of the digital systems allows both colour and monochrome pictures to be taken, viewed, and printed while the patient is with you. Treatment can then be started much sooner than would otherwise be possible.

# Virtual reality

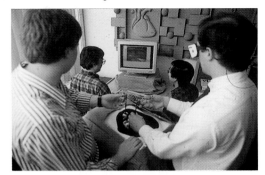

Practising an operation with virtual reality simulation.

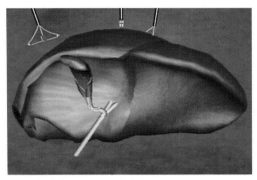

Screen image of a virtual liver.

The picture of practising an operation with virtual reality simulation is reproduced from J Coleman *et al*. *Br J Surg* 1994;81:1709–11, with permission of Blackwell Science. The picture of a virtual liver is reproduced with permission of Ciné-Med, Woodbury, Connecticut, USA.

Virtual reality refers to a computer generated representation of an environment that allows sensory interaction, thus giving you the impression that you are actually present. The immense complexity of human anatomy and the huge computational power needed to simulate it have so far limited the practical application of virtual reality technology in medicine. This technology has been most closely associated with the entertainment industry in the form of virtual reality video games.

The three ways of experiencing a virtual environment are through sound, sight, and touch. Virtual reality systems create a stereoscopic "visual immersion" by generating two slightly differing images that are alternately presented to each eye, giving the impression of a three dimensional image. This is usually achieved by positioning two small liquid crystal display (LCD) screens in front of each eye—a head mounted display.

## Medical applications

The simulation of realistic tactile and force feedback has been a major obstacle to the application of virtual reality systems in medicine. Currently virtual reality systems are being used in preoperative planning and training in minimally invasive surgery and have the potential to become powerful tools for teaching anatomy.

Computer generated simulators have been developed that allow images to be imported from computed tomography or magnetic resonance imaging. These permit an unparalleled view of anatomic structures previously accessible only by dissecting a cadaver. The advantage of this system is that it allows surgeons to plan and rehearse complex operations—such as reconstructive surgery or neurosurgery—before the patients ever reach theatre.

*Minimally invasive surgery*—Training in laparoscopic surgery has been under scrutiny after reports of serious complications. At present, initial training involves manipulating inanimate objects in purpose built training boxes. These allow the development of hand-eye coordination but lack anatomical detail and are therefore of limited use. A virtual reality simulator of laparoscopic cholecystectomy has been developed that allows a surgeon to practice manipulation of instruments and organ without compromising a patient's safety. The system resembles a conventional simulator but presents an anatomically correct image of the biliary system and allows organs to be grasped, retracted, and cut. The system is still at the prototype stage, but it has great potential for use in teaching and evaluating trainee surgeons. Another use for this system is in the design of new instruments before the manufacture of prototypes.

# 21   KEEPING YOUR COMPUTER HEALTHY AND LEGAL

**Routine maintenance tasks**

- Organise your hard disk
- Create a rescue floppy disk
- Backup your data
- Defragment the hard disk
- Scanning for viruses

Computers are generally very reliable, but failures can happen as a result of hardware breakdown, accidental deletion of an important file, virus infection, or simply unexplained corruption of your programs or data. In some organisations users can call on an IT department, but most people have no access to computer experts and have to try to fix problems themselves. Even an IT department may be unable to help unless you have taken a few basic precautions. Fortunately, there are many simple tasks that the ordinary user can do without special knowledge to protect the system and the data that it contains, and to minimise the risk of problems occurring in the first place.

## Organising your hard disk

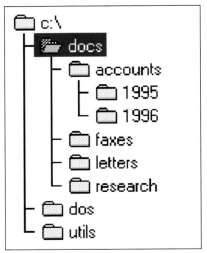

Organising your hard disk makes it easier to locate programs and data.

You should organise your hard disk properly so that programs and data can be located quickly and easily when they are needed. Starting at the C: \ prompt, create a series of new directories into which you put specific types of file. For example, you may wish to create a directory called C:\UTILS for utilities such as your text editor. To do this, either type md utils (make directory) at the DOS prompt or use Windows file manager and select File, Create Directory and then name it utils.

Create another directory called C:\DOCS for documents. You might then wish to create a series of subdirectories under C:\DOCS such as C:\DOCS\LETTERS or C:\DOCS\ACCOUNTS. Saving all your work in this way makes it much easier to back up your files, as you simply back up C:\DOCS and all its subdirectories, avoiding the need to locate a large number of word processor, spreadsheet, and database files scattered all over your hard disk. Programs should also be put into separate directories—most installation programs will automatically do this for you, but you may be prompted to choose a suitable name.

## Making a rescue disk

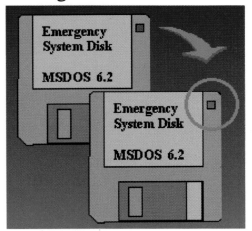

A rescue disk lets you get your computer back up and running in just a few minutes. When you have made one, slide the write protect tab to the open position to prevent other users (or a computer virus) from accidentally destroying it.

If your computer fails to start properly—perhaps because the hard disk has failed, because you have accidentally deleted an important file (such as command.com), or because a virus has corrupted the system—you will need a rescue disk to get the computer up and running so that you can investigate and correct the cause of the problem. To make a rescue disk, format a new floppy disk using the DOS command **Format a**: /s or use Windows file manager to create a system disk. Both methods copy the operating system on to the floppy disk.

It is a good idea to copy a few other essential files from the C:\DOS directory on to the disk, such as fdisk.exe, sys.com, format.com, and edit.com. These small programs allow you to prepare a completely new hard disk, or to wipe a corrupted one clean so that you can start again. You should also copy autoexec.bat and config.sys, which contain important configuration information specific to your computer. These files are modified from time to time (for example, when new programs are installed), so you should always keep an up to date copy. Do not forget to include a copy of your backup program, otherwise you will be unable to restore programs or data. Store your rescue disk in a safe place well away from stray magnetic fields such as those surrounding loudspeakers.

# Backing up your data

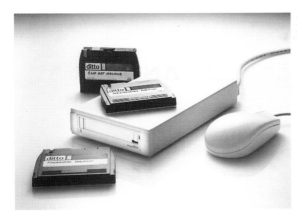

Tape streamers using the new Travan standard are capable of backing up very large hard disks (up to 3.2 gigabytes) on a single tape cartridge.

Most people keep just one copy of their work on their computer's hard disk. If the disk fails it can easily be replaced in a few minutes, but lost data often takes months or years to recreate and may even be irreplaceable. Records show that businesses which suffer such loss of data often become insolvent within a few months. To protect against this eventuality, all users should establish and regularly use a reliable backup system.

*Tape streamers*—The most convenient form of backup system is the tape streamer, which is capable of copying all the contents of the hard disk (operating system, directory structure, programs, and data) on to a single tape cartridge. Tape streamers are readily available, easy to install, and relatively cheap (although units capable of backing up very large, modern hard disks remain quite expensive). You should purchase and label a series of backup tapes so that a different one is used on each day of the week. It is also a good idea to make separate, monthly backup tapes and to keep old copies for a while because virus infections often take some time to become apparent—during which time your daily tapes may be storing infected programs.

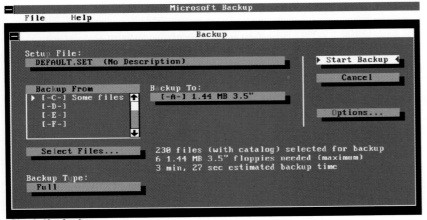

Microsoft's standard backup program is much better than simply copying files to floppy disks.

*Floppy disks*—Many users with relatively small amounts of data do not need the sophistication of a tape streamer as they can use floppy disks. A single high density floppy disk can, for example, store several hundred letters. Backup programs are usually capable of compressing your data files and allow you to store even more files on each disk. Nevertheless, feeding several floppy disks into the computer one after the other is time consuming and a disincentive to making regular backups.

MSDOS 6 includes a useful backup program, but it is limited to using floppy disks. Windows 95 includes a better one that also supports several different tape drives, and that can be run overnight or in the background while the computer is doing other work. More sophisticated programs are available and are often supplied free when you purchase a tape streamer.

*Freeing disk space*

Tape streamers can also be used to store little used programs or data, allowing you to delete them from your hard disk—making room for other software and possibly saving the need to purchase an additional or larger drive. A disadvantage is that these archived programs cannot be run from the tape and therefore need to be restored to the hard disk before they can be used again. An alternative approach is to use removable hard disk technology such as that produced by Iomega or Syquest. These removable disks operate just like a normal hard disk, though they tend to be slightly slower. The drives are more expensive than a standard hard disk drive, but the removable cartridges are relatively cheap and allow you to store an infinite number of programs or data. An additional advantage is that the cartridges can be removed from the computer and locked away in a safe overnight. Optical disks offer very high storage capacities and are robust, being immune to magnetic fields with a very long (50 year) life, but they remain expensive and are inappropriate for most situations.

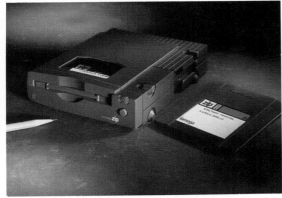

Removable hard disks can now store over 1 gigabyte of programs and data.

# Defragmenting your hard disk

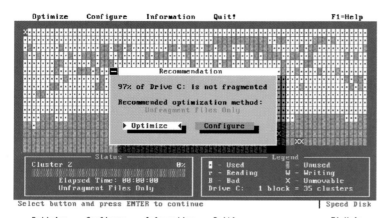

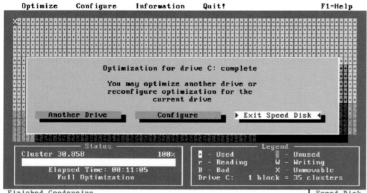

Badly fragmented hard disk, which slows the computer down (top), and same hard disk after running Norton Speed Disk (bottom).

When MSDOS stores a file on your hard disk, it looks for the first available free space and starts copying the file to that location. If the file is too large to fit in this space, DOS looks for the next bit of free space and stores part of the file there too, and so on. Large files can therefore end up badly fragmented. When you retrieve the file, DOS locates each fragment and reconstructs the original file. This is a slow process, and the mechanical parts of the hard disk are subjected to considerable wear as the heads move back and forth across the disk surface, increasing the risk of disk failure. Fragmentation becomes particularly important as your hard disk nears its maximum storage capacity.

To reduce fragmentation, you should regularly defragment your hard disk with a program such as Norton Speed Disk. This reorganises the contents of the hard disk so that the fragments are brought back together. It also allows frequently used files to be moved to the start of the disk, where they can be retrieved relatively quickly. A cut down version of Speed Disk (called defrag.exe) is given free with MSDOS 6. Defragmenting a large hard disk can take time, so it may be best to leave the program running overnight. Windows 95 automatically defragments the hard disk whenever it is necessary.

# Protecting your computer from viruses

## Common computer viruses

- Form (most common)
- Jack Ripper
- Antiexe
- Monkey2
- AntiCMOS
- Stoned
- Angelina
- Junkie
- Sampu
- Natas(Satan backwards)
- Telefonica

**The Michelangelo virus received an enormous amount of media attention recently but is only very rarely found to have infected computer systems.**

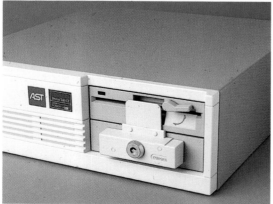

Mechanical devices to prevent insertion of floppy disks are an excellent defence against infection with a virus and unauthorised extraction of sensitive data.

Computer viruses are tiny programs designed to take advantage of the fact that computer users frequently exchange programs and data files on floppy disks and via modem links. A computer can be infected by a virus for many months or even years without you being aware of it, but at some predetermined date the virus will be activated. The effects of viruses range from mildly irritating messages on the screen to severe damage to your programs, data files, and even hardware. There are thousands of computer viruses, but most attacks are due to a relatively small number of common ones, such as the "form virus", which is currently responsible for about 80% of reported attacks (June 1995). Computer networks are also vulnerable: viruses first infect one workstation, but the infection soon spreads through the network to the file server and, from there, on to some or all of the other computers attached to the network.

### Protection

Fortunately, it is relatively easy to protect your computer by taking some simple precautions. Most viruses are acquired on infected floppy disks rather than by dialling into other computers with a modem. When an infected floppy disk is inserted into your computer the virus has an opportunity to copy itself on to your hard disk and to begin infecting your programs. Users who never share programs or data with others are most unlikely to acquire a computer virus. However, viruses have occasionally been found on the free disks on the front cover of computer magazines and even on original program installation disks, so it is prudent to treat all disks with suspicion. Before copying anything to or from a floppy disk that has been in another computer, run an up to date virus scanner to check that the disk is clear. Programs that have been downloaded via a modem should also be checked before they are run for the first time. Most scanners are also capable of safely removing viruses from a computer system, although it may still be necessary to reinstall your programs and to restore data from backups.

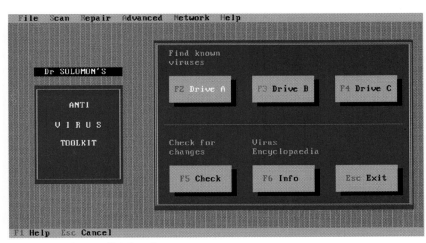

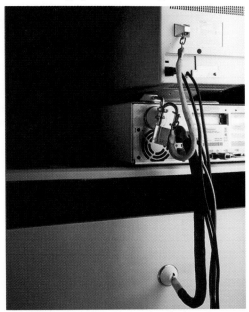

Scanning a floppy disk for viruses.

*Automatic scanning*—Virus scanners can be loaded into the computer's memory during booting up. These run continuously in the background, monitoring every program run on the computer, and give an instant warning if virus activity is detected. Most stop you from running infected programs by halting the computer. This type of scanner has the advantage of being totally automatic, but false alarms are not unknown and interfere with the smooth running of the system. Some computers have built in protection against certain types of virus affecting the boot sector of the hard disk. This feature is simple to activate by changing a setting in the computer's setup. However, it has been found to prevent installation of Windows 95 and should therefore be turned off before you upgrade the operating system (it can be safely turned on again afterwards).

# Protecting your computer from theft

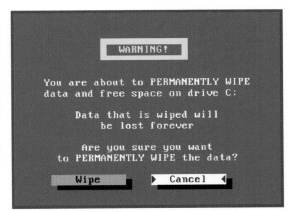

Securing your computer to the desk makes theft less likely—but does not stop theft of components such as RAM memory modules.

Computers are very attractive to thieves as it is easy to sell either whole machines or component parts such as memory modules that are small, valuable, and virtually untraceable. To reduce the risk, it is a good idea to indelibly mark the casing of the computer by engraving your name and postcode or by using an etching system such as Selectamark. Several companies sell devices that make it difficult to steal system boxes and monitors. Remember that the NHS does not insure its computer equipment, so good physical security measures are essential. One of the best deterrents is to lock the door of your surgery or office when you leave the room.

Many household insurance policies specifically exclude cover for home computers used for private practice, research, or other business purposes. Those which do are most unlikely to offer protection against financial losses incurred as a result of business interruption or the cost of restoring data to a new system. This problem can be solved by purchasing a home office insurance policy, which offers worldwide all risks cover for all your computer equipment (including portable computers, which are particularly vulnerable) at relatively modest cost. Serial numbers of your equipment should be recorded and sent to your insurance company.

# Securing your data

Norton WipeInfo permanently overwrites the data on your hard disk ensuring that it can never be retrieved.

Passwords are the most common way to restrict access to a computer system. Most IBM compatible machines can be set up so that a password is needed before the computer will start, but this can be defeated quite easily. Windows 95 offers somewhat better protection than MSDOS, but Windows NT is required for very tight security. Many programs (such as accounts or payroll packages) are password protected, and some word processors (such as WordPerfect) allow you to attach a password to individual files. Very secure systems which encrypt all the data on the disk are also available. If you leave a computer on line and set to answer the phone, it is vulnerable to hackers and you should take professional advice about measures such as automatic dial back.

Remember that deleting files from the hard disk does not remove the contents of the files but rather merely hides them and they can therefore be undeleted very easily. If you plan to sell a computer which has contained sensitive data it is essential to overwrite that data with a program such as Norton WipeInfo.

# Keeping within the law

## Eight basic principles of the Data Protection Act 1984

The act stipulates that data:

- Must be obtained and processed fairly and lawfully
- Must be held only for specified lawful purposes
- Must not be used in a manner incompatible with those purposes
- Must only be recorded where necessary for those purposes
- Must be accurate and up to date
- Must not be kept longer than necessary
- Must be made available to the patient on request
- Must be protected by appropriate security and backup procedures

## Useful sources of advice about computer security

| Organisation | Telephone No |
|---|---|
| Symantec (Norton Utilities) | 01628 592222 |
| S&S International (Dr Solomon's Anti Virus Toolkit) | 01296 318700 |
| McAfee Anti Virus (shareware) | 0171 631 0548 |
| Iomega | 0181 899 1734 |
| Europa Security | 01732 360573 |
| Tolson Messenger Insurance Brokers (home office policy) | 0800 374246 |
| Computer Crime Unit | 0171 230 1177 |
| Data Protection Registrar | 01625 545745 |

### Data Protection Act 1984

The data protection act applies to all computer systems that contain personal data relating to living people. It does not apply to paper based record systems. There are specific exclusions—such as data held by an individual in connection with personal, family, or household affairs or a practice's computerised payroll system—but all patient management systems including paperless health records must be registered with the Data Protection Registrar. These systems can, however, be used as soon as the application form is posted (that is, without waiting for approval, which may take up to six months).

People have the right to a written copy of the information which is held about them and to have inaccurate information corrected or erased. They also have a right to claim compensation if they suffer damage or loss as a result of inaccurate or lost data. Doctors have been granted the right to refuse to disclose information held about a patient if it would be likely to cause serious harm to his or her physical or mental health or if it would allow the patient to identify another person who has not consented to the disclosure of his or her identity. Comprehensive guidance notes on the act are available from the Data Protection Registrar and from the British Medical Association.

### Computer Misuse Act 1990

It is a criminal offence for an unauthorised person to access or attempt to access any part of a computer system, with or without intent to commit a serious crime such as theft, fraud, or blackmail; to carry out any unauthorised modification to programs or data (including the planting of viruses); or to prevent or hinder access to the system. These crimes carry severe penalties. Despite these deterrents, many computers are attacked by hackers each year. Anyone who suspects that their system has been tampered with or who finds a computer virus should notify the Computer Crime Unit, Scotland Yard.

### Health and Safety (Display Screen Equipment) Regulations 1992

These require all employers to assess computer workstations used by employees or self employed people on their premises in order to identify and minimise the various risks to which those people are exposed. There is an exemption for workstations that were already in use when the regulations came into force on 1 January 1993, but all workstations must comply by 31 December 1996.

The guide offers clear advice about who is considered a regular user (for example, medical secretaries) and who is not (for example, receptionists making only occasional use of the computer). Ergonomic factors such as seating position, neck posture, and glare from the screen as well as working patterns are covered in detail. Regular users are entitled to have their eyes tested on request at the employer's expense; if glasses prove to be necessary for work with the computer, these must be provided as well, although employers are not required to provide bifocals or expensive fashionable frames.

The aim of the regulations is to minimise the physical and mental stress associated with computer use. Careful attention to detail should reduce the risk of work related upper limb disorders (WRULD) and protect the employer from legal action for personal injury and breach of the law.

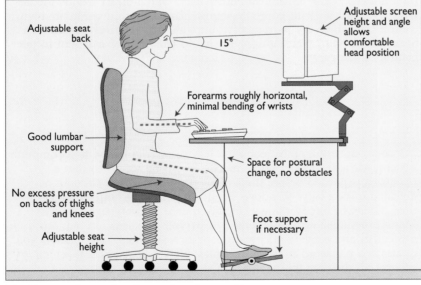

Ideal layout of a workstation and seating position.

# GLOSSARY

| | |
|---|---|
| Alt key | A key on either side of the spacebar which is used with other keys to activate quick commands |
| Anonymous FTP | A way of downloading files from a remote computer over the Internet without needing a password |
| ANSI | American National Standards Institute |
| ANSI.SYS | A file sometimes used in personal computers to control graphic displays |
| Archie | A program which can be used to search for files stored at FTP sites on the Internet |
| ASCII | American Standard Code for Information Interchange |
| ASCII File | A basic text file that has no formatting codes (e.g. bold, underline). Supported by all word processors |
| AT (ISA) bus | The pathway connecting internal components in all 286, 386 and some 486 computers |
| Attribute | Appearance applied to a character such as bold or italic |
| Auto-answer | A modem setting instructing it to automatically answer an incoming telephone call |
| Autoexec.bat | File read by DOS during the boot-up process. Contains configuration instructions |
| Background | Tasks being performed "out of sight" in a multitasking environment (eg background printing) |
| Backup | A duplicate copy of important programs or data files. Usually stored on tape or removable disks |
| Backward compatible | Something that allows you to continue using old (or obsolete) hardware or software |
| Bad sector | Area on a floppy or hard disk that is damaged and cannot be used to store data |
| Base font | The default font that is used throughout a document |
| Base memory | The first 640KB of random access memory |
| BASIC | Beginner's All-Purpose Symbolic Instruction Code. Easy to learn programming language |
| Batch file | A file containing a batch of DOS commands. Can be recognised by the file extension .BAT |
| Beta test software | Program that is undergoing evaluation prior to release of the final version |
| BIOS | Basic Input Output System. Set of programs that control the fundamental operation of a personal computer |
| Bit map | A bit map graphic is a picture composed of many tiny dots |
| Bold | A type that is heavier and darker than standard text |
| Boot disk | A floppy disk or hard disk containing an operating system |
| Boot up | The process that occurs immediately after switching on a computer during which the operating system is loaded from a boot disk leaving the computer ready for use |
| Break | A key which allows the user to pause the computer's operation |
| Bulletin board system (BBS) | A program run on a host computer that allows other users to dial in to leave messages for each other, read information on-line, and download shareware and public domain programs |
| BUS | The internal pathway along which various components of the computer communicate |
| BYTE | The fundamental unit of data storage—equivalent to just one character |
| C | High level programming language |
| Cache | An area of memory used to store recently used data which can be retrieved again very quickly if needed |
| Caps lock key | A key that locks the shift key—so that all letters appear in upper case |
| Centronics interface | A proprietary name for the parallel printing port |
| CHEST | Combined Higher Education Software Team. Negotiates competitive pricing deals |
| Clipboard | Used by programs to copy data both within and between documents |
| Clock speed | Term used to describe the speed at which the processor (CPU) operates |
| Cluster | A subdivision of the space on a hard disk which is created during formatting and contains a set number of bytes |
| Comma-delimited | A type of database file in which each piece of information in a record is separated by a comma |
| Command.com | Part of the operating system which translates plain English commands such as "COPY" into machine code |
| Compressed file | A file that has been reduced to a fraction of its original size without loss of data |
| Config.sys | File read by DOS during the boot-up process. Contains configuration instructions |
| Copy protection | Means by which illegal duplication of software is prevented |
| Corrupted file | A file which has become damaged. A file repair utility can sometimes repair it |
| CPU | Central Processor Unit. The chip that does most of the work in your computer |
| Crash | Term used when a program or sometimes the whole computer ceases to function |
| Cross-linked file | A corrupted file. Sometimes results from an error which occurs whilst saving a file to the hard disk |

# Glossary

| | |
|---|---|
| Ctrl Alt Del | One way to reboot the computer by simultaneously pressing these three keys |
| Ctrl key | Otherwise known as the control key. Used with other keys to activate quick commands |
| DDE link | Dynamic data exchange. Allows automatic exchange of data between two programs running simultaneously |
| Device driver | A small program that allows the computer to communicate with items such as printers and CD-ROMS |
| DIP switch | A small switch often found on expansion boards which is used to alter the board's configuration |
| DMA channels | Direct Memory Access Channels are used to transfer data from the computer's memory to other components |
| DOS | Disk Operating System. Synonymous with operating system |
| Download | Transfer of data or programs from a remote computer onto your hard disk |
| DPI | Dots per inch. Laser printers work at 300–600 dpi. Higher values give better print quality |
| Duplex printing | Printing on both sides of the paper without turning it over. Expensive option on some but not all printers |
| EIDE | Enhanced IDE standard that offers fast connection for up to four disk drives (including CD-ROM) |
| Email | Electronic mail. A way of sending messages to someone over a network or the Internet |
| Endnotes | Similar to footnotes but appear at the end of the chapter. |
| Escape codes | Codes used by a computer to control an attached printer |
| Ethernet | A type of network that uses coaxial cable to link computers to each other |
| Executable file | A program file which can be recognised by the extension .EXE or .COM |
| Expanded memory | One way of allowing DOS programs to use memory above the standard 640KB limit |
| Export | Term used when saving a document in anything other than the default file format |
| Extended memory | One way of allowing DOS programs to use memory above the standard 640KB limit |
| FAQ | Frequently asked questions |
| FAT table | File allocation table. An invisible record in which DOS stores details of the files on the hard disk |
| Fatal error | An error which occurs whilst running a program and from which recovery is not possible |
| Female connector | Has small sockets to receive the protruding pins of a male connector |
| Field | Space reserved for a single piece of information (e.g. surname) in a database record |
| File attribute | All files stored on personal computers have attributes such as R (read only), H (hidden), S (system) |
| File server | A central computer on a network used to store data and programs |
| Font | A collection of letters and numbers sharing a common typeface, point size and attributes (e.g. bold or italic) |
| Font cartridge | Added to a printer to expand the number of resident fonts. |
| Footer | User defined information (such as the title, author or page number) that automatically prints at the bottom of every page in a document |
| Formatting | Process that prepares a hard or floppy disk for use in a computer |
| FTP | File transfer protocol |
| Full justification | Process in which the spacing between words is automatically adjusted so that each line of text starts and ends at the margins |
| Function keys | Row of keys along the top of the keyboard labelled F1 to F12. Used to activate commands |
| GDI Printer | A low cost laser printer that takes advantage of the Windows environment to process the image prior to printing |
| GUI | Graphical user interface (such as Windows) |
| Handshake | Automatic process that occurs when two modems connect during which they negotiate optimal communication |
| Hard space | Prevents two words from being separated by automatic word wrapping at the end of a line of text |
| Hardware | The physical components of a computer system |
| Hardware reset | A way of completely restarting the computer by pushing the reset button on the front panel |
| Header | User defined information (such as the title) that automatically prints at the top of every page in a document |
| Hidden file | A file with a hidden attribute which remains invisible during a standard directory listing |
| Hypertext link | A highlighted word which, when clicked with a mouse, takes you automatically to another part of the document |

| | |
|---|---|
| ICON | A graphical symbol on the screen which represents a particular program or file |
| IDE | Standard interface that allows connection of one or two hard disks to the computer |
| Import | Term used when loading a file created by another program |
| Incremental backup | Backing up only those files that have changed since you last did a back up |
| I/O | Input/Output system—the link between the CPU and other components |
| IRQ | Interrupt ReQuest. Means by which peripherals signal that they are ready to send or receive data |
| ISA | Industry Standard Architecture |
| JANET | Joint Academic NETwork |
| JPEG | Joint Photographic Experts Group. Devised a compressed graphic file format which can be recognised by the extension .JPG |
| Jumper | Tiny connector which is placed onto pins on a circuit board, in order to select different configurations |
| Justification | Alignment of text along either the left or the right margin or around the centre line |
| Kernel | Core part of the operating system |
| Kerning | Adjustment of the space between letters in a word so that the spacing looks even |
| Landscape | Paper orientation with the longest edge horizontal |
| Light pen | Light sensitive pen that allows you to draw on a VDU and select functions by pointing to them |
| Line art | Graphic image containing just lines and no shading or colour. File size is usually very small |
| Local bus | Modern, high speed communications pathway that replaces the AT or ISA bus. There are various standards (VESA, MCA, and PCI) but the PCI bus is now dominant |
| Locked file | A file that has been password protected to prevent unauthorised access |
| Logical drives | All or part of a hard disk or a network drive that has been assigned a unique letter such as C: D: or E: |
| Login name | Unique name which you use along with a password to log into a computer system or network |
| Lost chain | Hard disk error in which there is an entry in the FAT table but the link to the file on the disk is lost |
| Lost cluster | Hard disk error in which there is no entry in the FAT table for the file on the disk |
| Macro | A way of performing a predetermined series of tasks within a program by pressing just one key |
| Mail merge | A process in which a letter template is merged with information from a database in order to create a series of customised letters |
| Mainframe | A very large computer that can handle several thousand users simultaneously |
| Male connector | Connector with protruding pins that connect into the corresponding sockets on a female connector |
| Margins | Points at the top, bottom or side of a page where printing starts or stops |
| Memory address | A specific location in your computer's random access memory |
| MIDI | Musical Instrumental Digital Interface. International protocol which allows computers to communicate with and control musical synthesizers |
| Monospaced font | Typeface such as courier in which each letter occupies the same amount of space. Commonly used in traditional typewriters |
| Multitasking | A way of running two or more programs simultaneously by sharing processor time between them |
| Network administrator | The person responsible for maintaining a network, issuing passwords etc |
| Newsgroup | A discussion group on a bulletin board system or the Internet |
| Newspaper column | Layout in which text flows down one column to the bottom then flows on to the next one along |
| Non-interlaced | A high quality monitor mode which minimises screen flicker |
| Null modem cable | A cable used for transferring data between two computers via their serial ports |
| Num lock key | Locks the numeric keypad into numeric entry mode |
| Numeric key pad | The cluster of keys on the right side of a keyboard which allows very fast entry of numerical data |
| OCR | Optical Character Recognition. A process in which a scanned picture of some text is "read" electronically resulting in a standard text file that can be indexed, saved or edited in a word processor |
| OEM | Original Equipment Manufacturer |
| Off-line | Refers to the time when a peripheral (eg modem or printer) is not communicating with the computer |
| OLE | Object Linking and Embedding. A dynamic data link between different programs |

# Glossary

| | |
|---|---|
| Operating system | The program (such as MSDOS, OS/2, Windows 95) which controls the basic operation of the computer |
| Outline font | A font that does not loose its quality when it is enlarged, unlike bit mapped fonts |
| Overwrite mode | Keyboard mode in which newly typed characters overwrite those already on the screen |
| Page break | Code embedded in a document which instructs the printer to start a new page at that point |
| Page preview | Allows the user to see exactly what the page looks like before it is printed |
| Parallel port | Socket found on the back of the computer which is usually used to connect a printer |
| Partition | A section of the data storage area on the hard disk |
| Path | List of directories in which DOS will look for program files after a command is issued |
| PCMCIA | Personal Computer Memory Card International Association who defined a type of expansion slot commonly found on portable computers into which you can plug very compact modems, network cards or hard disks. Recently been renamed PC card socket |
| PCX | Bit mapped graphics file format |
| Peripheral | A component connected to and controlled by the computer such as CDROM, tape streamer, modem or printer |
| PIM | Personal Information Manager. A program which organises and stores personal data |
| Plug and play | A system that allows you to simply plug in new components saving much time and effort although both the computer and the new component must support the standard for this to work |
| Point size | A term used to describe the size of a font |
| Polyline | A drawing tool using a number of straight lines to form a shape |
| Polycurves | A drawing tool using a number of curved lines to form a shape |
| Portrait | Paper orientation with the longest edge vertical |
| PostScript | A high quality printing language (can only be used with a PostScript printer) |
| Print spooler | A background printing utility which allows you to continue working on the computer whilst it is printing |
| Printer emulation | Allows a printer to behave like an older and more common model (such as laserjet II) so that it can be used with programs which do not support the latest standards |
| Proportional font | Typeface such as Times Roman in which letters occupy a variable amount of space depending their width |
| Query | Term for a detailed search through a database for very specific information |
| Quit | Leave an application. Common short cuts include alt-X, Esc and Alt-F4 (Windows) |
| RAM | Random-access memory. Working space in which instructions and data are stored prior to processing |
| RAM disk | A very fast but temporary disk drive created in RAM which can be used to speed up the computer's operation |
| Rasterisation | The process of producing a bit mapped image from a vector graphic |
| README.TXT | An ASCII text file found commonly on installation disks giving important additional information or help |
| Read-only file | A file with the read-only attribute set, which can be viewed but not altered or deleted |
| Reboot | Restart the computer |
| Refresh | Re-draw the image or text on the computer screen |
| Rendering | Converts line art into a solid three dimensional image |
| Reset button | Normally found on the front panel of the computer and is used to reboot the computer |
| RISC | Reduced Instruction Set Computer. A modern alternative to the 80X86 CPU design |
| ROM | Read Only Memory. Contents are not lost when the power is turned off but it is slower than RAM |
| Root directory | The first directory on a drive (on a hard disk usually termed C:\) |
| Scalable font | A font outline that can be enlarged to any size on the screen or printed page |
| Screen dump | Captures and prints the current image on the screen |
| Screen saver | A program that displays moving images after a period of inactivity in order to prevent damage to the screen |
| Script | A set of instructions that tell the computer how to perform complex tasks |
| SCSI | Small Computer System Interface. Allows you to connect up to seven SCSI devices such as hard disks, CDROM drives or a tape streamer in a daisy chain. Generally faster than IDE but complex to set up |
| Serial port(s) | Socket(s) found on the back of the computer usually used to connect mouse and modem |
| Serif font | A typeface, such as the one used here, in which there are small cross strokes on the letters making the text easy to read |
| Shadow RAM | A reserved part of RAM into which the computer places a temporary copy of the data normally stored in the relatively slow ROM thereby allowing much faster access to that data |
| Site licence | A licence to use multiple copies of a program within one office/building/company |

| | |
|---|---|
| Snail mail | Term used when referring to the standard postal service |
| Soft font | A typeface stored on the hard disk and only downloaded to the printer as needed |
| Software licence | Document that gives the right to use a program but which does not normally confer ownership of it |
| Software piracy | Illegal duplication of copyrighted software |
| Sound board | An expansion card that allows the computer to play high quality sound |
| Sub-directory | A directory below the root directory such as C:\WINDOWS or C:\DOS |
| SYSOP | System Operator. The person who maintains a bulletin board system |
| Tab-delimited file | A type of database file in which each piece of information in a record is separated by a tab |
| TCP/IP | Transfer Control Protocol/Internet Protocol. The method of communication used on many networks including the Internet |
| TIFF | Tagged Image File Format. A bit mapped graphic file format |
| Terminal | A combination of keyboard and screen which is used to access and control a distant computer |
| Terminal emulator | Program that allows a computer to behave like a dumb terminal |
| Text file | A file containing just standard ASCII characters with no formatting information |
| Thread | A term used in newsgroups to indicate a series of linked messages |
| Thumbnail | A small, low resolution, representation of a much larger graphic image. Useful for finding the right picture |
| TIFF | Tagged Image File Format. A bit mapped graphic file format your work |
| Toolbar | A row of buttons that activates short cuts in a program. Normally found at the top of the screen |
| Touch screen | Pressure sensitive monitor screen. Can be used instead of a mouse |
| Trackball | An alternative to the mouse favoured by some people |
| TSR | Terminate-and-stay-resident program which is loaded into RAM at bootup and remains there, ready for use, without delay until the computer is switched off |
| UAE | Unrecoverable application error. Sometimes seen when a Windows program has crashed |
| UNIX | An 32 bit, multiuser operating system commonly found on Internet servers and GP computer systems |
| Undo | Undoes the last command |
| Upgrade | Conversion of an existing program to the latest version usually at a discount compared to the retail price |
| Upload | Transfer of data or programs from your hard disk onto a remote computer |
| Upper memory | Area of memory between base 640KB and 1MB |
| UPS | Uninterruptible power supply. Protects important systems by ensuring a continuous power supply |
| VDU | Video display unit or monitor |
| Vector graphics | A method of creating and saving an image by describing its outline. These images can be enlarged to any size without degradation (unlike bit mapped images) |
| VESA | Video Electronics Standards Association |
| VGA | Video Graphics Array. A high resolution display standard used in monitors. Most modern computer systems and monitors now support an enhanced version called super VGA (sVGA) |
| Video card | The interface card that collects digital signals from the processor and drives the screen |
| Visual basic | A programming language used to create Windows applications |
| VRAM | Video RAM. Very fast but expensive memory specially designed for high performance video cards |
| Wild card | A * character used in search strategies (e.g. DIR *.BAT would list all files ending with that extension) |
| WMF | Windows Metafile Format. A vector graphics file format |
| Word wrapping | Process in which any text that extends beyond the right margin is automatically moved down onto the next line. |
| WORM | Write Once, Read Many times. An optical storage device ideal for audit trails |
| Write back cache | A cache that delays saving information on the hard disk until the computer is idle |
| Write protect | A way of preventing the computer overwriting valuable information on a disk |
| Write through cache | A cache that saves information on the hard disk immediately but retains a copy for fast access if required |
| WWW | World Wide Web. Pages of graphical information on the Internet joined to each other by hypertext links |
| WYSIWYG | What You See (on the screen) Is What You Get (on the paper) |
| ZIF socket | Zero Insertion Force Socket. A socket that allows easy insertion and removal of the CPU when required |

# INDEX

# Index

# ABCs from the BMJ

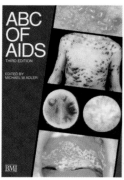
ISBN 0 7279 0761 1

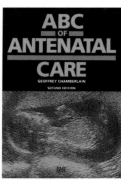
ISBN 0 7279 0884 7

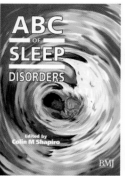
ISBN 0 7279 0794 8

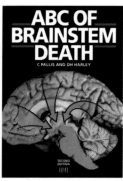
ISBN 0 7279 0245 8

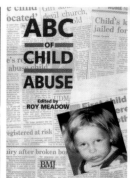
ISBN 0 7279 0764 6

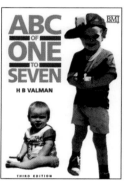
ISBN 0 7279 0768 9

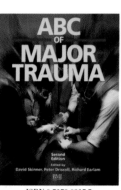
ISBN 0 7279 0917 7

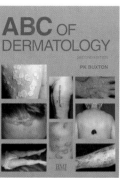
ISBN 0 7279 0777 8

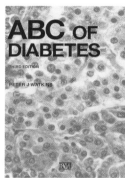
ISBN 0 7279 0763 8

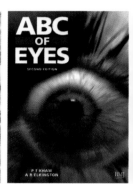
ISBN 0 7279 0766 2

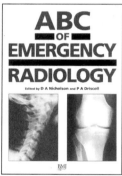
ISBN 0 7279 0832 4

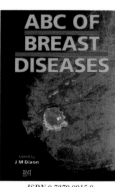
ISBN 0 7279 0915 0

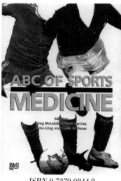
ISBN 0 7279 0844 8

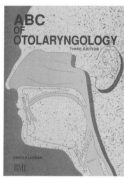
ISBN 0 7279 0765 4

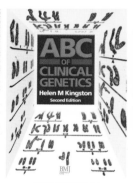
ISBN 0 7279 0846 4

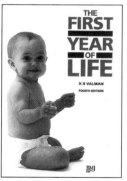
ISBN 0 7279 0897 9

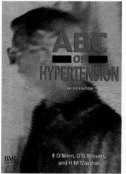
ISBN 0 7279 0769 7

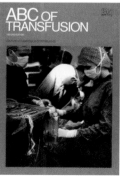
ISBN 0 7279 0754 9

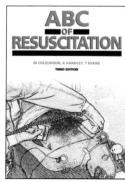
ISBN 0 7279 0839 1

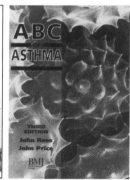
ISBN 0 7279 0882 0

**For further details contact your local bookseller or write to:**

BMJ Publishing Group
BMA House
Tavistock Square
London WC1H 9JR  (U.K.)

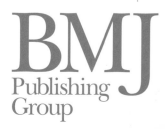

BMJ
Publishing
Group